T0227233

Polypharmacy

Editors

EDWARD SCHNEIDER
BRANDON K. KORETZ

CLINICS IN GERIATRIC MEDICINE

www.geriatric.theclinics.com

November 2022 • Volume 38 • Number 4

ELSEVIER

1600 John F. Kennedy Boulevard • Suite 1800 • Philadelphia, Pennsylvania, 19103-2899

http://www.theclinics.com

CLINICS IN GERIATRIC MEDICINE Volume 38, Number 4
November 2022 ISSN 0749–0690, ISBN-13: 978-0-323-96197-4

Editor: Taylor Hayes
Developmental Editor: Hannah Almira Lopez

Clinics in Geriatric Medicine (ISSN 0749-0690) is published quarterly by Elsevier Inc., 360 Park Avenue South, New York, NY 10010-1710. Months of issue are February, May, August, and November. Business and Editorial Offices: 1600 John F. Kennedy Blvd., Suite 1800, Philadelphia, PA 191023-2899. Periodicals postage paid at New York, NY, and additional mailing offices. Subscription prices are $303.00 per year (US individuals), $712.00 per year (US institutions), $100.00 per year (US & Canadian student/resident), $330.00 per year (Canadian individuals), $901.00 per year (Canadian institutions), $431.00 per year (international individuals), $901.00 per year (international institutions), and $195.00 per year (international student/resident). Foreign air speed delivery is included in all *Clinics* subscription prices. All prices are subject to change without notice. POSTMASTER: Send address changes to *Clinics in Geriatric Medicine,* Elsevier Health Sciences Division, Subscription Customer Service, 3251 Riverport Lane, Maryland Heights, MO 63043. **Telephone: 1-800-654-2452 (U.S. and Canada); 314-447-8871 (outside U.S. and Canada). Fax: 314-447-8029. E-mail:** journalscustomerservice-usa@elsevier.com **(for print support)** or journalsonlinesupport-usa@elsevier.com **(for online support).**

Reprints. For copies of 100 or more, of articles in this publication, please contact the Commercial Reprints Department, Elsevier Inc., 360 Park Avenue South, New York, New York 10010-1710. Tel.: 212-633-3874; Fax: 212-633-3820, E-mail: reprints@elsevier.com.

Clinics in Geriatric Medicine is covered in *MEDLINE/PubMed (Index Medicus), EMBASE/Excerpta Medica, Current Contents/Clinical Medicine (CC/CM),* and the *Cumulative Index to Nursing & Allied Health Literature.*

Contributors

EDITORS

EDWARD SCHNEIDER, MD
Professor of Gerontology, Medicine and Biology, Emeritus Dean of the Andrus Gerontology Center, USC Leonard Davis School of Gerontology, Los Angeles, California

BRANDON K. KORETZ, MD, MBA
Carol and Jim Collins Endowed Chair, Professor of Clinical Medicine, David Geffen School of Medicine at UCLA, Los Angeles, California

AUTHORS

ASAL M. AZIZODDIN, PharmD
Department of Medicine, Division of Hematology/Oncology, UCLA David Geffen School of Medicine, Los Angeles, California

ALBERT BUI, MD
Advanced Primary Care Program, Geriatric Medicine, High Risk Medical Director, PIH Health Hospital, Whittier, California

WYNNELENA C. CANIO, MD, CMD, AGSF
Chief of Geriatric Medicine, Kaiser Permanente San Rafael, San Rafael, California

KIMBERLY Y. CHEN, DO
Primary Care, Welbe Pacific/PACE, Pasadena, Geriatric Medicine Fellow, Keck School of Medicine, Los Angeles, California

JUSTIN J. CHENG, MD
Department of Medicine, Wake Forest School of Medicine, Winston-Salem, North Carolina

HELEN CHERNICOFF, MD
Fellow, Combined Geriatrics and Palliative Care, Division of Geriatrics, Department of Internal Medicine, Hospice and Palliative Medicine Program, University of California, Los Angeles, Los Angeles, California

CHARLES EDWARD COFFEY JR. MD, MS
Clinical Associate Professor of Medicine, Keck School of Medicine of USC, Los Angeles, California

ERIN ATKINSON COOK, MD
Associate Professor of Clinical Medicine, UCLA Department of Medicine, Division of Geriatrics, Los Angeles, California

ESTEBAN COTA, MD
Fellow, Department of Geriatric Psychiatry, University of California, Los Angeles, Los Angeles, California

ANALIESE DICONTI-GIBBS, MD
Clinical Assistant Professor of Medicine, Division of Geriatrics, Hospital, Palliative, and General Internal Medicine, Keck School of Medicine of USC, Los Angeles, California

MARIA DUENAS, MD
Geriatric Medicine Fellow, UCLA Department of Medicine, Division of Geriatrics, Los Angeles, California

MANUEL A. ESKILDSEN, MD, MPH
Clinical Professor, Department of Internal Medicine, Division of Geriatrics, University of California, Los Angeles, Los Angeles, California

PATRICIA HARRIS, MD, MS
Professor of Clinical Medicine, UCLA Department of Medicine, Division of Geriatrics, Los Angeles, California

LAURA A. HART, PharmD, MS
Health Sciences Assistant Clinical Professor, Skaggs School of Pharmacy and Pharmaceutical Sciences, University of California, San Diego, La Jolla, California

JASON JALIL, MD
Department of Psychiatry and Biobehavioral Sciences, Semel Institute for Neuroscience and Human Behavior, University of California, Los Angeles, Los Angeles, California

JASON P. LEE, MD
Fellow, Department of Geriatric Psychiatry, University of California, Los Angeles, Los Angeles, California

RUTH MADIEVSKY, PharmD
Clinical Pharmacist, Division of General Internal Medicine and Health Services Research, University of California, Los Angeles, Los Angeles, California

MICHAEL J. MARANZANO, MD
Department of Medicine, Division of Hematology/Oncology, UCLA David Geffen School of Medicine, Los Angeles, California

MEGAN MCCONNELL, MD
Division of Endocrinology, Diabetes, and Metabolism, Department of Medicine, UCLA David Geffen School of Medicine, Los Angeles, California

PARGOL NAZARIAN, PharmD, BCPP
Department of Pharmacy, Stewart and Lynda Resnick Neuropsychiatric Hospital, University of California, Los Angeles, Los Angeles, California

KHAI H. NGUYEN, MD, MHS
Health Sciences Associate Clinical Professor, Department of Medicine, University of California, San Diego, La Jolla, California

ELAINE ROH, MD
Fellow, Geriatric Medicine, Department of Internal Medicine, Division of Geriatrics, University of California, Los Angeles, Los Angeles, California

NARINE SARGSYAN, PharmD
Department of Medicine, Division of Hematology/Oncology, UCLA David Geffen School of Medicine, Los Angeles, California

JOHN SHEN, MD
Department of Medicine, Division of Hematology/Oncology, UCLA David Geffen School of Medicine, Los Angeles, California

ALBERT SHIEH, MD
Assistant Professor, Division of Endocrinology, Diabetes, and Metabolism, Department of Medicine, UCLA David Geffen School of Medicine, Los Angeles, California

AMY Z. SUN, MD
Fellow, Combined Geriatrics and Palliative Care, Department of Internal Medicine, Division of Geriatrics, Hospice and Palliative Medicine Program, University of California, Los Angeles, Los Angeles, California

VAISHAL TOLIA, MD, MPH
Professor, Department of Emergency Medicine, University of California, San Diego, La Jolla, California

HANS F. VON WALTER, MD
Division of Geriatric Mental Health, Department of Psychiatry, Greater Los Angeles VA Healthcare System, Los Angeles, California

ANGELA YEH, DO
Division of Geriatrics, Assistant Clinical Professor, Department of Internal Medicine, Hospice and Palliative Medicine Program, University of California, Los Angeles, Los Angeles, California

Contents

> Polypharmacy, associated with adverse health outcomes, is common in older adults owing to increasing chronic conditions. In addition to normal organ system changes that affect pharmacokinetic, and pharmacodynamics of medications, drug-drug interaction and drug-disease interactions should be reviewed. Tools to minimize polypharmacy should be considered when treating older adults.

> Although hypertension is highly prevalent in older adults, treatment goals require both an understanding of the various guidelines available, as well as appreciation of the unique medical, cognitive, psychosocial, and functional heterogeneity of our individual geriatric patients that may place them outside those guidelines. As a patient's clinical status changes over time, clinicians may consider deprescribing their blood pressure medications when their risks begin to outweigh their benefits. Unique clinical circumstances and incorporating the time to benefit of hypertension control help guide clinical decision-making.

> Behavioral and psychological symptoms of dementia (BPSD) may occur in most patients with dementia. Symptoms such as agitation, aggression, and psychosis often lead to higher rates of hospitalization, morbidity, and mortality. Despite the prevalence of BPSD, safe and effective treatment options are limited. This often leads to off-label prescribing and trends toward polypharmacy. Notwithstanding modest efficacy in BPSD, antipsychotics seem to be one of the most commonly prescribed medications in its treatment. Polypharmacy with antipsychotics is particularly troublesome due to the increased risk of potentially lethal adverse effects. As such, their use should be judiciously monitored with the goal of gradual dose reduction.

comorbidities. Polypharmacy is influenced by drug–drug interactions and can reduce the efficacy of systemic cancer therapeutics. It is also associated with worse progression-free and overall survival for some cancers such as lung and colorectal cancer. This highlights the need for a judicious review of all medications and the role of interventions in improving quality of life and survival.

In older adults, polypharmacy and osteoporosis frequently occur contemporaneously. Polypharmacy is increasingly recognized as a risk factor for hip and fall-related fractures. Treatments for osteoporosis include antiresorptive (alendronate, risedronate, zoledronic acid, ibandronate, denosumab) and osteoanabolic (teriparatide, abaloparatide, romosozumab) agents. Polypharmacy is associated with worse adherence to pharmacologic therapy. Thus, the selection of osteoporosis treatment should be individualized and based on a variety of factors, including underlying fracture risk (high vs very high risk), medical comorbidities, medication burden, as well as fracture risk reduction profiles, modes of administration, and side effects of treatment options.

Polypharmacy in the emergency department (ED) presents additional challenges for older adults with acute illnesses but is also an opportunity for healthcare providers to prevent adverse drug events as well as the use of potentially inappropriate medications. Older patients have complex health-related needs and are at risk for medication-related complications during an ED visit. Implementing mitigating strategies of performing medication reconciliation and review, using existing implicit or explicit tools to evaluate medications, and deprescribing or de-escalating high-risk medications are critical to positive health outcomes. These practices can help to optimize pharmacologic interventions for older patients in the ED.

CLINICS IN GERIATRIC MEDICINE

SERIES OF RELATED INTEREST

Primary Care: Clinics in Office Practice
https://www.primarycare.theclinics.com/
Immunology and Allergy Clinics
http://www.immunology.theclinics.com/

THE CLINICS ARE AVAILABLE ONLINE!
Access your subscription at:
www.theclinics.com

Preface

Polypharmacy: A Continuing Challenge to Clinicians

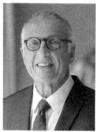

Edward Schneider, MD   Brandon K. Koretz, MD, MBA
Editors

We, clinicians, took an oath to cause no harm. One of the most common ways that clinicians can cause harm is by through prescribing unnecessary medications and/or prescribing medications that interact negatively with other medications.

DEFINITION

There have been many definitions of polypharmacy. Masnoon[1] tabulated 138 definitions of polypharmacy, of which 111 used a numerical definition. The most common number was five or more medications. Some made the important distinction of appropriate versus inappropriate or problematic medications.[2] Rather than number of medications, the definition that we favor for polypharmacy is the use of one or more unnecessary or inappropriate medications, since, in our opinion, that is the real issue. Beers, from that small college in Westwood, came up with classifying inappropriate medications. We believe that prescribing inappropriate medications is probably more worrisome than the absolute number of medications.

WITH AGING, THERE IS INCREASED COMORBIDITY WITH RESULTANT INCREASES IN MEDICATION NUMBERS

Chronic conditions increase in frequency with aging.[3] Therefore, it is not surprising that the number of prescribed medications increases with aging and that polypharmacy is a significant issue in older patients.

MEDICINE IN THE UNITED STATES IS PROVIDED IN SILOS, WHICH INCREASES THE RISK OF POLYPHARMACY

Health care silos may provide efficient care for specific conditions, but often the health care providers in these silos do not take the time to address all the medications the

Clin Geriatr Med 38 (2022) xi–xiii
https://doi.org/10.1016/j.cger.2022.07.010
0749-0690/22/© 2022 Published by Elsevier Inc.

patient may be prescribed by doctors in other silos. As a result, the patient is at risk of polypharmacy with potential drug-drug interactions.

THE NUMBER OF MEDICATIONS PRESCRIBED FOR SENIORS IS INCREASING

From 1988 to 2018, the percent of Americans using five or more prescription drugs increased from 4% to 11%.[4] For those ages 65 years and older, the percent exploded from 13.8% to 41.9% during this same time. There were no significant differences by sex. There were some differences by ethnicity with older Asian Americans and Hispanic/Latino Americans having the lowest percent, 6.6%, and African American elders having the highest percent of taking five or more prescribed medications at 12.4%.

IN AMERICA, POLYPHARMACY IS PROFITABLE

Pharmaceutical companies in the United States are raking in the dollars. On average, Americans spend twice as much ($1126 per capita) than their peers in other countries on prescription medications ($552).[5]

POLYPHARMACY INCREASES WITH AGING

Three-quarters of those ages 50 to 65 years used prescription drugs compared with 91% of those ages 80 years and above. Even more importantly, the number of drugs prescribed increases from 13 at ages 50 to 64 years to 22 for those ages 80 years and above.[6] The tragedy is that more than half of the prescription costs for those 65 years and above is out of pocket, and for those ages 80 years and over, this percent increases to 67%.

POLYPHARMACY LEADS TO INCREASING PROBLEMS WITH COMPLIANCE, ADVERSE DRUG RESPONSES, AND DRUG-DRUG INTERACTIONS

With more medications prescribed to a patient, the risk of compliance, adverse drug responses, and drug-drug interactions increases.

POLYPHARMACY IS NOT JUST PRESCRIPTION DRUGS

Older Americans, accounting for just 13% of the US population, purchase 40% of all over-the-counter (OTC) medications.[7] These OTC medications include treatments for allergies, upper respiratory infections, arthritis, heartburn, and constipation.[7] More that 3 million Americans reported using herbal remedies.[6] The supplement to the NHIS 2002 included questions related to alternative medications, and 12% had used them.[8,9]

DEPRESCRIBING AS A RESPONSE TO POLYPHARMACY

One of us (E.L.S.) was at the National Institutes of Health, leading an initiative for reducing polypharmacy that featured television and radio interviews. After one of these interviews, E.L.S. received a call from a nursing home administrator who proudly told me that he was stopping all the medications to his older residents. We must be careful to emphasize the importance of appropriate medications while we reduce polypharmacy.

Edward Schneider, MD
USC Leonard Davis School of Gerontology
1946 North Serrano Avenue
Los Angeles, CA 90027, USA

Brandon K. Koretz, MD, MBA
David Geffen School of Medicine at UCLA
200 UCLA Medical Plaza, Suite 420
Los Angeles, CA 90095, USA

E-mail addresses:
eschneid@usc.edu (E. Schneider)
BKoretz@mednet.ucla.edu (B.K. Koretz)

REFERENCES

1. Masnoon, Shakib S, Kalisch-Ellet I, et al. What is polypharmacy? A systematic review of definitions. BMC Geriatrics 2017;17:230–40.
2. Payne RA. The epidemiology of polypharmacy. Clin Med 2016;16:465–9.
3. Marengoni A, Angleman S, Melis R, et al. Aging with multimorbidity: a systematic review of the literature. Ageing Res Rev 2011;10(4):430–9.
4. Centers for Disease Control and Prevention. Table 39. Prescription drug use in the past 30 days, by sex, race and Hispanic origin, and age: United States, selected years 1988-1994 through 2015-2018. Available at: https://www.cdc.gov/nchs/data/hus/2019/039-508.pdf. Accessed date May 16, 2022.
5. Kurani N, Kurani N, Cotliar D. How do prescription drug costs in the United States compare to other countries? Peterson-KFF Health System Tracker. Available at: https://www.healthsystemtracker.org/chart-collection/how-do-prescription-drug-costs-in-the-united-states-compare-to-other-countries/#Per%20capita%20prescribed%20medicine%20spending,%20U.S.%20dollars,%202004-2019. Accessed date May 16, 2022.
6. Georgetown University. Prescription drugs. Health Policy Institute. Available at: https://hpi.georgetown.edu/rxdrugs/. Accessed date May 16, 2022.
7. Berardi RR, Kroon LA, McDermott JH, et al. Handbook of nonprescription drugs: an interactive approach to self-care. 15th edition. Washington DC: American Pharmacist Association; 2006. p. 5.
8.. Wilheim M, Ruscin JM. The use of otc medications in older adults. US Pharm 2009;34(6):44–7.
9. Arcury TA, Grzywacz JG, Bell RA, et al. Herbal remedy use as health self-management among older adults. J Gerontol B Psychol Sci Soc Sci 2007;62(2):S142–9.

Polypharmacy in Older Adults

Wynnelena C. Canio, MD, CMD, AGSF*

KEYWORDS

- Older adults • Basic pharmacology • Prescribing cascade • Polypharmacy
- Potentially inappropriate medications • Deprescribing

KEY POINTS

- Polypharmacy, associated with adverse health outcomes, is common in older adults owing to increasing chronic conditions.
- In addition to normal organ system changes that affect pharmacokinetic, and pharmacodynamics of medications, drug-drug interaction and drug-disease interactions should be reviewed.
- Tools to minimize polypharmacy should be considered when treating older adults.

INTRODUCTION

As a result of continued advancement in medicine, more people are living longer. In 2014, there were 46.3 million Americans (14.5%) who were at least 65 years old. This number is projected to more than double to about 98 million (23.5%) by 2060.[1] More drugs, including nutraceuticals, are available each year, and Food and Drug Administration and off-label indications of drugs are expanding. Although this age group comprises about 15% of the US population, the members collectively account for 33% of all prescription medication use and 40% of nonprescription medication use.[2] Older adults usually have chronic conditions that require some treatment. In 2012, 60% of older adults were being treated for 2 or more chronic conditions.[3] Per evidence-based guidelines, these conditions are usually treated with multiple medications; the result is polypharmacy. For instance, if one is diagnosed with diabetes mellitus, current guidelines may include one or more glucose-lowering drugs to meet a certain glycemic control, the use of aspirin for primary prevention of cardiovascular disease, and treatment of comorbid hypertension and hyperlipidemia.

The prevalence of polypharmacy is reported to be between 10% and 90%, a wide range owing to different definitions of polypharmacy, age groups, and geographic locations.[4] In a systematic review of related terms, 138 definitions of polypharmacy

Kaiser Permanente San Rafael, 1650 Los Gamos, Suite 270 W, San Rafael, CA 94903, USA
* Corresponding author.
E-mail address: Wynnelena.C.Canio@kp.org

Clin Geriatr Med 38 (2022) 621–625
https://doi.org/10.1016/j.cger.2022.05.004
0749-0690/22/© 2022 Elsevier Inc. All rights reserved.

geriatric.theclinics.com

were found.[5] The most widely accepted definition of polypharmacy is the use of 5 or more medications per day.[6] As illustrated in earlier discussion, some comorbidities require the use of multiple medications and may be appropriate for some patients. These medications have improved health and life expectancy of older adults. However, polypharmacy has been associated with increased risk of adverse health outcomes, drug interactions, hospitalizations, and medical costs.[7] Patients with multiple comorbidities are particularly at risk, especially during transitions of care. They can also be a victim of prescription cascade. To minimize these risks, clinicians must be mindful of treatment options discussed with patients, including reviewing over-the-counter (OTC) medications and supplements, considering what matters most to the patients, which is usually preserving function and independence, and being especially attentive to potentially inappropriate medications.

BASIC PHARMACOLOGY AND AGING

Aging is associated with changes in the function of various organ systems and receptors, increasing sensitivity to drug effects in older adults.[8] An older adult prescribed with benzodiazepine may experience more sedation and poorer psychomotor skills. Amount absorbed is not changed, but absorption may be slowed with aging. Drugs that reduce gastrointestinal motility, such as antihistamines, can change the absorption of other drugs.[8] As one ages, fat stores increase and lean body mass decreases, which cause a relative increase in the volume of distribution of fat-soluble drugs, such as most central nervous system (CNS) active drugs. Increases in the fat to lean body mass ratio can lead to higher blood levels of medications, such as morphine, levodopa, or lithium. There is also slower glomerular filtration rate and hepatic blood flow, which reduces clearance of many drugs. Drug metabolites with long half-lives can accumulate over time and lead to toxic effects. All of these changes can increase the risk for adverse drug reactions (ADRs), such as falls, orthostatic hypotension, bleeding, renal failure, and delirium. About 5% to 28% of acute geriatric medical admissions are due to ADRs.[9] Most ADRs (95%) are considered predictable.[9] ADRs can usually be offset by a decrease in dosing rate, using smaller doses and/or longer intervals such that the total dose per unit time is lower. This is the basis for the "start low and go slow" mantra in geriatric prescribing. Even if this is followed, the increased number of drugs used in older adults may still cause unpredictable response, because of drug-drug interactions.

DRUG-DRUG INTERACTIONS IN OLDER ADULTS

Drug-drug interactions are common in older adults. The risk increases as more medications are prescribed, especially if there are multiple physicians treating the patient. Older adults might take a drug that inhibits, or induces, the metabolism of other medications. Many older adults receive a combination of drugs that can affect cytochrome P450 (CYP) function, with results in clinically important interactions.[10] Although CYP 3A activities appear to be reduced with aging, the phase II process of glucuronidation is somewhat affected by aging but may be affected by body habitus, smoking, and certain disease states.[11] Not surprisingly, the risk of a drug-drug interaction increases with the number of drugs a patient takes. This risk is 13% for patients taking 2 medications and 82% for patients taking more than 6 medications.[12] The risk of potential adverse drug interactions increases as new medications are added for new acute conditions for those people who are already taking several medications. Serious drug-drug interactions usually involve medications with narrow therapeutic indices, such as digoxin, antiarrhythmic, warfarin, and central-acting analgesics.

DRUG-DISEASE INTERACTIONS

Drug-disease combinations can affect drug response and lead to ADRs. Sometimes, it can exacerbate existing conditions. This drug-disease interaction has been observed in as many as 15% of older adults.[13] The most common observed interactions were the use of first-generation calcium channel blockers in patients with congestive heart failure and the use of aspirin in patients with peptic ulcer disease in one study.[13] It has also been shown that patients with dementia can have increased sensitivity or paradoxic reaction to CNS active drugs. As discussed earlier, clearance of many drugs is slowed down with aging alone, so patients with kidney and hepatic failure may be at increased risk for drug toxicity.

PRESCRIBING CASCADE

Prescribing cascade can affect any age, but it is more common in older adults owing to their use of multiple medications. Prescribing cascade is defined as occurring when signs and symptoms of an adverse drug event are misinterpreted as a new medical condition and a new treatment is further added to treat the adverse drug event.[14] An example of this is a 75-year-old man diagnosed with mild-stage Alzheimer disease who was prescribed donepezil, a cholinesterase inhibitor. At 5 mg, he was observed to be more attentive, although he started having urinary incontinence and diarrhea at 10 mg. The prescribing physician was out of the office when these symptoms were shared. A covering physician prescribed oxybutynin for urinary incontinence and dicyclomine for the diarrhea. This patient ended up in the emergency room for worsening confusion with visual hallucinations. Despite being identified, the prescribing cascade as shown is increasing in our health systems and should be addressed owing to potential risks and costs.

POTENTIALLY INAPPROPRIATE MEDICATIONS
Anticholinergics

Acetylcholine, a neurotransmitter, activates both nicotinic and muscarinic receptors. Anticholinergics are a class of medications that block the acetylcholine in the brain and peripheral tissues. They are prescribed for and used by older adults for several medical conditions. About 11.4% of those 65 years old and older have been prescribed anticholinergic drugs as compared with 3.8% of younger adults.[15] Two or more anticholinergic drugs were used in 32% of older adults living in nursing homes and 13% of those living at home.[16] Use of anticholinergics is associated with anticholinergic burden, measured in several ways that consider number, dose, and/or degree of anticholinergic activity of medicines.[17] This has been shown to be a predictor of adverse health and functional outcomes, so this should be minimized, if possible.[16] Older adults are at increased risk of anticholinergic toxicity. Symptoms that may suggest central anticholinergic toxicity include restlessness, irritability, agitation, confusion, disorientation, hallucinations, tremor, seizures, sedation, and coma.[18]

Central Nervous System Drugs

As previously mentioned, older adults are more susceptible to the effects of CNS acting drugs, such as antidepressants, muscle relaxants, opioids, antipsychotics, and benzodiazepines, because of age-related changes in pharmacology. Many older adults take these drugs to treat common conditions, such as osteoarthritis, depression, and sleep disorders.[18] Older adults taking one or more sedating medications are at increased risk for cognitive impairment and falls.[18] When combined, these drugs have an additive effect.

Over-the-Counter Remedies

More than 300,000 OTC medications are available today.[19] These medications are usually used to self-medicate common conditions, such as upper respiratory symptoms, insomnia, pain, heartburn, constipation, and oral, skin, and eye care.[19] They are generally considered safe for the general population but carry risks in older adults, and if used more than the recommended period of time. Some of these medications have ingredients that have anticholinergic properties (such as diphenhydramine in OTC medications for allergies, cold, and sleep aids) that may be inappropriate, as illustrated above. Some OTC medications may interact with other medications. For instance, nonsteroidal anti-inflammatory drugs, such as ibuprofen, may cause bleeding ulcers, increase blood pressure, and cause acute kidney failure for those with existing kidney conditions and heart failure.

OPTIMIZING PRESCRIBING

Safe and effective medication use is crucial in caring for older adults. Polypharmacy-reducing strategies should be implemented. To treat any conditions, "start low and go slow," adjusting the dose based on renal or hepatic function and reviewing for possible medication and disease interaction. Review for any duplication or nonpharmacological treatment. Any new signs or symptoms should be considered a side effect of any recently prescribed or stopped medications or supplements before starting a new medication to treat the new condition. Nonadherence to medications may appear to be a poor response, which may further add another medication to meet treatment goal. Several tools have been designed to help reduce polypharmacy in older adults. These tools include American Geriatrics Society (AGS) Beers criteria[20] and Screening Tool of Older Persons' Prescriptions/Screening Tool to Alert to Right Treatment (STOPP/START).[21] It is always important to engage the patient when implementing deprescribing.

SUMMARY

Reducing inappropriate polypharmacy will help improve care in the increasing complex needs of older adults. In addition to routine review of current medications and nutraceuticals, knowledge of basic pharmacology in aging, drug-drug and drug-disease interactions, and tools, such as AGS Beers and STOPP/START, will help optimize prescribing.

DISCLOSURE

The author has nothing to disclose.

REFERENCES

1. Colby SL, Ortman JM. Projections of the size and composition of the U.S. population: 2014 to 2060, current population reports, P25-1143. Washington (DC): U.S. Census Bureau; 2014.
2. Shah BM, Hajjar ER. Polypharmacy, adverse drug reactions, and geriatric syndromes. Clin Geriatr Med 2012;28:173–86.
3. Ward BW, Schiller JS, Goodman RA. Multiple chronic conditions among US adults: a 2012 update. Prev Chronic Dis 2014;11:130389.
4. Khezrian M, McNeil CJ, Murray AD, et al. An overview of prevalence, determinants and health outcomes of polypharmacy. Ther Adv Drug Saf 2020;11.

5. Masnoon N, Shakib S, Kalisch-Ellett L, et al. What is polypharmacy? A systematic review of definitions. BMC Geriatr 2017;17(1):230.
6. Bjerrum L, Rosholm J, Hallas J, et al. Methods of estimating the occurrence of polypharmacy by means of prescription database. E J Clin Pharmacol 1997; 53:7–11.
7. Davies LE, Spiers G, Kingston A, et al. Adverse outcomes of polypharmacy in older people: systematic review of reviews. J Am Med Dir Assoc 2020;21:181–7.
8. Turnheim K. Drug dosage in the elderly. Is it rational? Drug Aging 1998;3:357–79.
9. Medina-Walpole A, Pacala JT, Potter JF. Geriatric syllabus. 9th edition 2016. p. p106.
10. Sandson NB. Appendix A. P450 tables. In: Drug interaction casebook. The cytochrome P450 system and beyond. Washing (DC): American Psychiatric Publishing; 2003. p. 251–69.
11. Liston HL, Markowitz JS, DeVane CL. Drug glucuronidation in clinical psychopharmacology. J Clin Psychopharmacol 2001;21:500–15.
12. Goldberg RM, Mabee J, Chan L, et al. Drug-drug and drug-disease interactions in the ED: analysis of a high-risk population. Am J Merg Med 1996;14(6):447–50.
13. Lindblad CI, Hanlon JT, Gross CR, et al. Clinically important drug-disease interactions and their prevalence in older adults. Clin Ther 2006;28:1133–43.
14. Rochon PA, Gurwitz JH. The prescribing cascade revisited. Lancet Lon Egl 2017; 389(10081):1778–80.
15. Remillard AJ. A pharmacoepidemiological evaluation of anticholinergic prescribing patterns in the elderly. Pharmacoepidemiol Drug Saf 1998;5:155–64.
16. Blazer DG, Federspiel CF, Ray WA, et al. The risk of anticholinergic toxicity in the elderly: a study of prescribing practices in two populations. J Gerontol 1983; 38:31–5.
17. Nishtala PS, Salahudeen MS, Sarah H. Anticholinergics: theoretical and clinical overview. Expert Opin Drug Saf 2016;15:753–68.
18. Hayes BD, Klein-Schwartz W, Barrueto F. Polypharmacy and the geriatric patient. Clin Geriatr Med 2007;23-2:371–90.
19. Safari D, DeMarco EC, Scanlon L, et al. Over-the-Counter Remedies in older adults. Clin Geriatr Med 2022;38:99–118.
20. American Geriatrics Society 2019 Updated AGS Beers Criteria for Potentially Inappropriate Medication Use in Older Adults. J Am Geriatr Soc 2019;67(4): 674–94.
21. O'Mahony D, O'Sullivan D, Byrne S, et al. STOPP/START criteria for potentially inappropriate prescribing in older adult: version 2. Age Ageing 2015;44:213–8.

Polypharmacy in Hypertension

Should Hypertensive Therapy Be Re-evaluated Periodically?

Albert Bui, MD*

KEYWORDS

- Hypertension • Deprescribing • Time to benefit • SPRINT trial • JNC-8

KEY POINTS

- Hypertension (HTN) treatment goals in older adults require consideration of their multimorbidities, unique clinical, psychosocial and functional circumstances, overall prognosis, and goals of care.
- Deprescribing HTN medications should include a discussion with patients on its risks versus benefits, medication tapering schedules required, and close follow-up over weeks and months to determine their net effect.
- Time to benefit of HTN control helps guide clinicians on assessing polypharmacy and deprescribing decisions for older adults.

Abbreviations	
SNRI	Serotonin and norepinephrine reuptake inhibitor
DASH	Dietary Approaches to Stop Hypertension
BID	twice daily
TID	3 times daily
PRN	as needed
TIA	Transient ischemic attack

INTRODUCTION

Hypertension (HTN) is commonplace in the geriatric population and is present in 76% of adults aged 65 to 74 years and in 82% of adults aged older than 75 years.[1] HTN is categorized into 4 categories by systolic blood pressure (SBP) and diastolic blood pressure (DBP) levels per the 2017 American College of Cardiology and American Heart Association task force:

- Normal blood pressure (BP): less than 120/less than 80 mm Hg

Advanced Primary Care Program, Geriatric Medicine, PIH Health Hospital, Whittier, CA, USA
* 12522 Lambert Road, Whittier, CA 90606.
E-mail address: albert.bui@pihhealth.org

Clin Geriatr Med 38 (2022) 627–639
https://doi.org/10.1016/j.cger.2022.05.005
0749-0690/22/© 2022 Elsevier Inc. All rights reserved.

Table 1
List of hypertension practice guidelines

Study/Guideline	Recommended Blood Pressure Goal	Notes
SPRINT	SBP goal <120 mm Hg	Age 50 y or higher
SPRINT SENIOR	SBP goal <120 mm Hg	Age 75 y or older
2014 JNC-8	BP < 150/90, age >60 y BP < 140/90, age <60 y	
STEP trial	SBP 110–130 mm Hg	Age 60–80 y
ACP	SBP <150 mm Hg SBP <140 mm Hg with cerebral vascular accident/TIA	Age 60 y or older
2017 ACC/AHA	BP < 130/80	Age 65 y or older
2020 ISH guidelines	SBP <140 mm Hg acceptable SBP <130 mm Hg ideal	

Abbreviations: ACC, American College of Cardiology; ACP, American College of Physician; AHA, American Heart Association; ISH, International Society of Hypertension Global Hypertension Practice Guidelines; JNC-8, Joint National Committee-8; SPRINT, Systolic Blood Pressure Intervention Trial; STEP, Strategy of Blood Pressure Intervention in the Elderly Hypertensive Patients.

- Elevated BP: 120 to 129/less than 80 mm Hg
- HTN Stage 1: 130 to 139 or 80 to 89 mm Hg
- HTN Stage 2: greater than 140 or greater than 90 mm Hg

Although patients are traditionally defined as having HTN when their SBP is more than 120 or their DBP is more than 90 on 2 separate readings, these cutoffs may not always be appropriate for geriatric patients. Certainly, the control of HTN aims to reduce end-organ damage (ie, myocardial infarction, left ventricular hypertrophy, renal dysfunction, stroke, and so forth) but clinicians also face the dilemma of potential side effects, such as presyncope or syncope, falls, pill burden, and more. Weighing these risks versus benefits becomes increasingly pertinent in geriatric patients where providers must consider their patients' multimorbidities, frailty, and cognitive impairment. Numerous studies[2–7] provide some guidelines in BP goals but clinicians are challenged to sort through these guidelines and determine if they apply to their specific patient population. For example, should we target lower SBP less than 120 according to the Systolic Blood Pressure Intervention Trial Senior trial[5] or tolerate higher BP < 150/90 for individuals older than 60 years according to Joint National Committee-8 (JNC-8)[3]? **Table 1** lists additional studies and their BP targets.

Limitations of Study Guidelines

Although many of these studies appropriately evaluated older adults, capturing the entire heterogeneity of the geriatric population is challenging. Applying these study results to particular patients with a wide variety of medical, cognitive, and psychosocial backgrounds may not always be appropriate. For example, the SPRINT trial excluded study participants with prior stroke, dementia, diabetes, nursing home patients, reduced left ventricular ejection fraction (<35%), and nonambulatory patients. Additionally, BP measurement was performed after the patient was seated for 5 minutes at rest, which is a standard that may not be met consistently in the outpatient setting. The inclusion and exclusion criteria for these studies are helpful in guiding clinicians in BP target goals but are also inherently limited in application to all patients.

DIFFERENTIAL DIAGNOSIS

Primary vs Secondary HTN: Primary HTN, or essential HTN, is the most common form of HTN in older adults. Secondary HTN, which is HTN due to an underlying cause, such as obstructive sleep apnea, renal artery stenosis, hyperaldosteronism, thyroid disorders, cortisol disorders, or pheochromocytoma are less common and beyond the scope of this article. However, clinicians should consider secondary HTN causes when BP control remains poor despite being on 3 or more maximally dosed medications, or if the patient's clinical history is concerning for these other causes.

Other Considerations in Difficult to Control Hypertension May Include

- White coat HTN
- Improper BP measurement technique
- Nonadherence to the treatment plan

Drugs, Certain Foods, and Over-the-Counter Supplements May Also Contribute to hypertension, Including

- Caffeine in energy drinks, coffee, teas
- Alcohol
- Nonsteroidal anti-inflammatory drugs
- Pseudoephedrine found in over-the-counter (OTC) allergy medications
- Anticholinergics, such as diphenhydramine (Benadryl), found in allergy and sleeping pills
- Street drugs (ie, cocaine, amphetamines)
- Nicotine products (ie, cigarettes)
- Glucocorticoids (ie, prednisone)
- St. John's wort
- Saw palmetto
- Licorice
- Headache medications, including ergotamine or caffeine-containing formulations
- Psychotropics
  - Serotonin and norepinephrine reuptake inhibitor (SNRI)—venlafaxine
  - Antipsychotics—clozapine, olanzapine

TREATMENT GUIDELINES

When BP control is desired, regardless of the specific BP goal, clinicians may offer both lifestyle and pharmacologic recommendations to their patients.

Lifestyle Interventions

- *Weight loss and diet:* The vast array of weight loss and diet options is beyond the scope of this article but clinicians are often asked for their opinions on various fad diets and nutrition recommendations. These diets include Dietary Approaches to Stop Hypertention (DASH) diet, low salt, calorie restriction, intermittent fasting, keto diet, paleo diet, Mediterranean diet, plant-based diet, whole foods diet, starch diet, and many more. Although there is growing literature on the benefits of various diets, it remains challenging to recommend any one-size-fits-all approach, especially in the geriatric population where multimorbidity, frailty, unintentional weight loss, cognitive, and swallowing function complicate overall goals.

- *Exercise*: Both aerobic and strength training exercises are highly encouraged to maintain functional independence along with reducing cardiovascular risk. However, physical limitations often pose challenges for geriatric populations to engage fully. These limitations include:
  - ○ Joint and muscle pain
  - ○ Spinal stenosis
  - ○ Prior stroke
  - ○ Deconditioning
- *Behavioral*: Stress management is increasingly recognized as an important aspect of health, and interventions include meditation, yoga, and biofeedback.

Pharmacologic Interventions

First-line pharmacologic treatments include 4 main drug classes, including diuretics, angiotensin-converting enzyme inhibitors (ACE-I) and angiotensin II receptor blockers (ARBs), calcium channel blockers (CCBs), and beta blockers. **Table 2** provides a list of common monotherapy and combination formulations.

Second-line options include vasodilators and alpha blockers.

Monotherapy versus combination therapy

Clinicians may initiate a single BP medication and titrate up to its maximum dose in order to reach the desired BP target goal. However, for patients who have difficulty controlling BP or inability to tolerate drug side effects, combining 2 BP medications may be more effective than monotherapy.[8–14] For example, combination benazepril plus hydrochlorothiazide or amlodipine was better than benazepril monotherapy. Furthermore, combination therapy at lower doses may be more effective than monotherapy at max doses in controlling BP. However, drug cost coverage and available formularies may limit therapy options.

Although younger patients or those with less comorbidities may tolerate any of these medications, older adults with increasing multimorbidities may be less resilient to potential side effects and require a more cautious approach. Indeed, personalizing pharmacologic treatment becomes increasingly important for older adults, and recognizing unique circumstances may guide clinicians on choosing appropriate therapies.

PHYSICAL EXAMINATION: CONSIDERATIONS IN POLYPHARMACY

Traditionally, the main objectives of the physical examination are to evaluate for potential secondary causes of HTN (ie, obstructive sleep apnea, renal artery stenosis, and so forth), end organ damage (ie, fundoscopic examination and other cardiovascular disease), as well as laboratory (ie, lipids, fasting glucose, electrolytes, renal function, thyroid hormone) or radiology testing (ie, chest X-ray, echocardiogram).

However, additional evaluation may be useful in evaluating polypharmacy in older adults:

Orthostatic vitals: Although orthostatic hypotension may occur at any age, older adults may have more exaggerated BP fluctuations and delayed recovery, increasing the risk of falls and injury. Obtaining orthostatic vitals requires measuring BP and heart rate readings in 3 different positions, lying, sitting and standing, and allowing roughly 2 to 5 minutes in between readings. Orthostatic vitals are considered positive if:

- SBP reduces by 20 mm Hg or more
- DBP reduces by 10 mm Hg or more

Positive orthostatic vitals must also incorporate associated symptoms, such as lightheadedness, weakness, vision changes, and syncope. Interpretation of these

Table 2
List of common blood pressure medications, including monotherapy and combination therapies

	Drug Class	Drug	Dose	Frequency
First-line therapies	Thiazide diuretics	Hydrochlorothiazide (HCTZ)	12.5–25 mg	Daily
		Chlorthalidone	6.25–25 mg	Daily
	ACE-I	Lisinopril	2.5–40 mg	Daily
		Benazepril	10–40 mg	Daily
		Captopril	6.25–50 mg	bid or tid
		Enalapril	2.5–40 mg	Daily
	ARB	Losartan	25–100 mg	Daily
		Olmesartan	20–40 mg	Daily
		Valsartan	80–320 mg	Daily
	CCB; dihydropyridines	Amlodipine	2.5–10 mg	Daily
		Nifedipine	30–90 mg	Daily
		Felodipine	2.5–10 mg	Daily
	CCB; nondihydropyridines	Verapamil	40–360 mg	tid
		Diltiazem	60–360 mg	bid
	Beta blocker	Metoprolol tartrate (short-acting)	12.5–100 mg	bid
		Metoprolol succinate (long-acting)	25–100 mg	Daily
		Carvedilol	3.125–25 mg	BID
		Bisoprolol	2.5–10 mg	Daily
		Atenolol	25–100 mg	Daily
Second-line therapies	Vasodilators	Hydralazine	10–200 mg	bid or tid
		Isosorbide mononitrate	20–120 mg	Daily
	Alpha-1 blockers	Terazosin	1–20 mg	Daily or bid
		Doxazosin	1–16 mg	Daily
		Prazosin	1–20 mg	bid or tid
	Alpha-2 adrenergic agonist	Clonidine	0.1–1.2 mg	bid
		Clonidine patch	0.1–0.3 mg	Weekly
	Loop diuretics	Furosemide	10–160 mg	Daily – qid
		Bumetanide	0.5–4 mg	Daily – tid
		Torsemide	2.5–50 mg	Daily
	Aldosterone antagonist	Spironolactone	25–100 mg	Daily
	Potassium-sparing diuretic	Triamterene	25–100 mg	Daily
	Direct renin inhibitor	Aliskiren	150–300 mg	Daily

(continued on next page)

Table 2
(continued)

Drug Class		Drug	Dose	Frequency
Combination therapies	Diuretic combinations	Amiloride and HCTZ	5 mg/50 mg	
		Spironolactone and HCTZ	25 mg/50 mg, 50 mg/50 mg	
		Triamterene and HCTZ	37.5 mg/25 mg, 50 mg/25 mg, 75 mg/50 mg	
	Beta blocker and diuretics	Atenolol and chlorthalidone	50 mg/25 mg, 100 mg/25 mg	
		Bisoprolol and HCTZ	2.5 mg/6.25 mg, 5 mg/6.25 mg, 10 mg/6.5 mg	
		Metoprolol and HCTZ	50 mg/25 mg, 100 mg/25 mg, 100 mg/50 mg	
		Propranolol and HCTZ	40 mg/25 mg, 80 mg/25 mg	
	ACE-I and diuretics	Benazepril and HCTZ	5 mg/6.25 mg, 10 mg/12.5 mg, 20 mg/12.5 mg, 20 mg/25 mg	
		Enalapril and HCTZ	5 mg/12.5 mg, 10 mg/25 mg	
		Lisinopril and HCTZ	10 mg/12.5 mg, 20 mg/12.5 mg, 20 mg/25 mg	
	ARB and diuretics	Losartan and HCTZ	50 mg/12.5 mg, 100 mg/25 mg	
		Valsartan and HCTZ	80 mg/12.5 mg, 160 mg/12.5 mg	
	CCB and ACE-I	Amlodipine and benazepril	2.5 mg/10 mg, 5 mg/10 mg, 5 mg/20 mg	
		Diltiazem and enalapril	180 mg/5 mg	
		Felodipine and enalapril	5 mg/5 mg	
	Triple therapy pill	Telmisartan	20 mg	
		Amlodipine	2.5 mg	
		Chlorthalidone	12.5 mg	
		Olmesartan	20–40 mg	
		Amlodipine	5–10 mg	
		HCTZ	12.5–25 mg	
		Amlodipine	5–10 mg	
		Valsartan	160–320 mg	
		HCTZ	12.5–25 mg	
	Quadruple therapy pill	Irbesartan, amlodipine, HCTZ, atenolol	37.5 mg/1.25 mg/6.25 mg/12.5 mg	

Abbreviations: ACE-I, angiotensin-converting enzyme inhibitor; ARB, angiotensin II receptor blocker; CCB, calcium channel blocker.

signs of symptoms should consider any multimorbidities or polypharmacy that may confound the clinical picture; see section "Unique challenges in the older adult" for more examples.

Cognitive examination: Patients with signs or symptoms of cognitive impairment warrant further evaluation of any potential reversible causes, such as polypharmacy. The various causes of cognitive impairment include age-related cognitive decline, mild cognitive impairment, dementia due to various causes (ie, Alzheimer vs Lewy Body vs vascular, and so forth) or encephalopathy due to a multitude of causes. Mood disorders may also affect cognitive function. Cognitive screening tools include:

- Mini-cog
- Animal naming
- Trails A&B
- Mini mental status examination
- Montreal Cognitive Assessment
- Rowland Universal Dementia Assessment Scale
- Confusion Assessment Method
- Geriatric Depression Scale
- Patient Health Questionnaire 9

These screening tools aim at assessing multiple cognitive domains, including executive decision-making, orientation, impulse control, short-term recall, attention, language, and mood. Selection of the most appropriate screening tools is also important and should consider a patient's cultural, language, and educational backgrounds.

The clinician should pay special attention to any medications with anticholinergic properties that may impair cognition (see more details in section "Unique Challenges in the older adult"). A diagnosis of cognitive impairment from any cause may have implications on BP goals. For example, a patient with end-stage dementia with dysphagia and falls likely has a poor overall prognosis and would be unlikely to benefit from tight BP control. Additional examples are provided in section "Unique Challenges in the older adult."

Gait and balance examination: Evaluating a patient's gait and balance are important in evaluating potential BP medication polypharmacy and their risk in falls and injury. Useful gait and balance tools include:

- Timed Up and Go Test
- Tinetti Gait and Balance Assessment
- 4-Stage Balance Test

A patient with poor balance or a history of frequent falls may benefit from reducing BP medications.

UNIQUE CHALLENGES IN THE OLDER ADULT

Although clinicians have numerous treatment guidelines for various diseases, patients with multimorbidities often have treatments that directly counter and conflict with those same guidelines. As a result, both clinicians and patients are sometimes offered opposing recommendations. Below are several examples of unique challenges in treating BP:

- *Pill burden*: Adherence becomes an issue when more prescriptions and OTC supplements are taken. Financially, copays and out-of-pocket expenses make affordability of various medications troublesome. For patients requiring caregiver support, keeping track of pill administration adds further challenges. Daily versus bid or tid or qid dosing complicate adherence. Altogether, patients may sometimes miss several doses per day or week and make both BP and other disease control inconsistent and substandard.

- *Dysphagia*: Dysphagia becomes an increasing barrier to medication adherence. In neurodegenerative diseases, such as Alzheimer dementia, Parkinson dementia, or stroke, oropharyngeal dysphagia tends to develop, which consequently affects patients' ability to adhere to oral medications. Alternative formularies such as subcutaneous injections or transdermal patches might allow some substitutions but cost and feasibility may be limiting factors. Feeding tubes are also considered to administer oral meds but have their own risks.[15,16] Specifically, feeding tubes (gastrostomy or G-tubes) used in patients with dementia increases risk of complications, such as agitation, infections, need for physical or pharmacologic restraints, and pressure wounds; altogether, quality of life diminishes and mortality increases.

- *Parkinson disease, autonomic dysfunction, and labile blood pressures*: Labile BPs are a common occurrence in Parkinson disease due to both autonomic dysfunction and possible side effects of their dopaminergic treatments. Patients may paradoxically be placed on BP-lowering medication while also on PRN BP-elevating (ie, midodrine), leading to a complicated and difficult pendulum swing of BP control.

- *Cerebral vascular accident with orthostasis*: Although BP control is crucial as primary and secondary prevention for strokes, supratherapeutic control may be similarly deleterious leading to orthostatic hypotension and falls and injury.

- *Congestive heart failure (CHF) with orthostasis*: Similar to primary and secondary prevention for strokes, CHF treatments may also lead to presyncope or syncopal events leading to falls and injury.

- *Worsening renal function*: Although BP medications are standard treatments to prevent, slow down, and preserve renal function, these same medications may lead to acute kidney injury if not monitored regularly. Furthermore, older adults also have higher risks of inadvertently taking other nephrotoxic medications, poor hydration, or hospitalizations where renal function can worsen acutely.

- *Diuretics in liver cirrhosis and baseline hypotension*: Patients with end-stage liver disease often have baseline low BP due to vasodilatory and perfusion changes. However, these patients also take diuretics to manage their third spacing lower extremity edema and ascites, which may lead to both kidney injury and/or worsening hypotension.

- *Beta blocker and donepezil*: Alzheimer disease prevalence increases with age, and donepezil is commonly prescribed as a first-line pharmacologic treatment to slow down its progression. However, although procholinergic mechanism of action of donepezil may assist with a patient's cognition, it can also lead to bradycardia by activating the parasympathetic "rest and digest" system. Therefore, individuals on both beta blockers and donepezil must be monitored for bradycardia, hypotension, and presyncope symptoms.

- *Anticholinergic burden*: Anticholinergic burden refers to the cumulative effect of using multiple medications with anticholinergic properties. Although diphenhydramine is the classic anticholinergic medication known to cause anticholinergic toxidrome (ie, confusion, cognitive impairment, tachycardia, flushing, bowel changes, and so forth) in overdose cases, several BP medication can contribute to anticholinergic burden.[17] For example, ACE-I such as captopril, beta blockers, and loop diuretics, such as furosemide, all have mild anticholinergic properties, and when taken concomitantly may cause toxidrome side effects. Below are further examples of cardiac-related medications with anticholinergic properties

Cardiac-Related Medications with Anticholinergic Properties

- Atenolol
- Captopril
- Coumadin
- Digoxin
- Dipyridamole
- Disopyramide phosphate
- Furosemide
- Hydralazine
- Isosorbide
- Metoprolol
- Nifedipine
- Triamterene
- *Geriatric syndromes*: Geriatric syndromes describe a constellation of signs and symptoms that represent multiple organ system impairment. Examples include:
  - Dementia
  - Frailty
  - Incontinence
  - Falls
  - Weight loss

Patients with these geriatric syndromes are highly vulnerable to medication side effects, less resilient to their negative impacts, and take longer to recover from stress.

- *Psychotropics and dementia*: Psychotropics, such as trazodone, antipsychotics, serotonin norepinephrine reuptake inhibitors such as venlafaxine, and benzodiazepines can lead to unpredictable orthostatic and labile BPs and may warrant adjusting their other BP medications.

Unique Challenges During the COVID-19 Pandemic

- *Access to care and telemedicine during the COVID-19 pandemic*: At the time of this article writing, the coronavirus 2019 (COVID-19) pandemic has upended traditional medical practice, where telemedicine has become an increasingly crucial part of health-care delivery. Although telemedicine has provided health-care providers and patients valuable avenues of communication, care that requires in-person visits may be delayed. For example, monitoring medication side effects with a physical examination or laboratory may be limited, delayed, and suboptimal in telemedicine. Certainly, the use of better technology (ie, smart tablets and phones) or ancillary staff (ie, home health nurses) may help but cannot replace the in-person visit.
- *Access to care and patient reluctance during the COVID-19 pandemic*: Patient reluctance to come into the office poses another barrier to standard care, let alone HTN management. Many patients fear the spread of COVID-19, especially in waiting rooms, offices, ER and hospital buildings, and laboratory sites. As a result, evaluation may be delayed. Although increasing COVID-19 vaccination rates have dramatically reduced infection rates and alleviated patient fears, COVID-19 variants continue to pose future risk and may reinforce this reluctance to access care in a timely manner.

Refractory Hypotension

If patients remain symptomatically hypotensive despite tapering down medications, clinicians may consider additional interventions, such as:

- Increase hydration
- Increase sodium intake
- Compression stockings
- Abdominal binders
- Pharmacologic, such as midodrine or fludrocortisone

Certainly, these considerations must be weighed against complicating their existing comorbidities. For example, increasing fluid intake for a patient with liver cirrhosis may worsen their third-spacing edema, and so these interventions may be limited.

DISCUSSION

Overall, these examples illustrate the unique challenges that clinicians must consider when prescribing or deprescribing BP medications. Clinicians should periodically re-evaluate the benefit versus risk of BP medications.

Uncertainty in Geriatrics

Although guidelines such as JNC-8 and the SPRINT Senior trial provide a helpful framework for clinicians in treating HTN in older adults, the unique medical, cognitive, functional, and psychosocial domains of our geriatric patients are difficult to measure and often excluded in these studies. Because these domains become increasingly more complicated, the certainty of the benefits seen in these studies become less certain. Uncertainty is a common feature in caring for geriatrics, and clinicians are challenged to have a level of comfort with uncertainty.

Time to Benefit

Clinicians caring for geriatric patients may consider the time to benefit (TTB)[18] for any particular intervention, that is, how long it would take to benefit from a medication or procedure, especially when considering a patient's life expectancy. Although an alternative biostatistic measurement, number needed to treat, also may guide clinicians on the impact of a particular treatment or test, TTB helps to further individualize our care to a patient's unique circumstances. For patients, they may ask, "Will I benefit from this treatment?" or perhaps more importantly, "When will it help?" In treating HTN, the TTB may be 1 to 2 years. So, patients with less comorbidities and longer life expectancy beyond 2 years might be more suitable for more intensive BP goal, whereas individuals with shorter life expectancy might do better tolerating much higher BP levels. For these patients, the trade-off between taking fewer medications and tolerating higher BP goal becomes more pertinent as they become sicker or when a more palliative course is desired. Alternatively, a patient suffering from orthostasis may gain more balance and function off BP medications who is willing to accept a higher BP goal.

Deprescribing

Deprescribing is the intentional act of tapering down and removing previously prescribed medications. One might consider deprescribing a medication linked to a known complaint or side effect from a patient. For example, clinicians might recommend deprescribing a patient's diuretic first if they also complain of incontinence or nocturia. **Table 3** provides further examples:

Tapering Schedules

As clinicians consider deprescribing BP meds, there is no gold standard method in tapering doses. The typical half-life of common BP medications (ie, diuretics, ACE-I,

Table 3
Comparing hypertension drug classes and potential reasons to deprescribe

Medication	Reason to Deprescribe
Diuretics	• Incontinence • Cramps • Potassium supplements • Electrolyte disturbance (ie, hyponatremia) • Acute kidney injury
ACE-I/ARB	• Cough • Olfactory or gustatory impairment • Acute kidney injury
Calcium channel blocker	• Leg swelling
Beta blockers	• Cognitive impairment • Mood disorder
Overall class effects	• Presyncope/syncope • Falls • Dizziness • Balance • Weakness • Unintentional weight loss

ARBs, CCB, Beta blockers) are on the order of hours to days, so it is reasonable to expect changes in BP measurements to be reflected over days to weeks on dose adjustment. On a practical level, weekly or monthly follow-ups either with the clinician or with nursing or pharmacy staff is appropriate. Quicker tapers, such as on a weekly basis, may be preferable depending on the clinical scenario, such as a patient with frequent syncopal events. Slower tapers, such as over months, may be appropriate when a particular BP medication still has a known benefit and the clinician hopes to balance that benefit while reducing the known risks. For example, a patient on diuretics for both HTN and CHF who also complains of urinary incontinence may reduce their medications more slowly in order to avoid compromising their volume status.

It is important to set clear expectations when deprescribing. A medication taper is a trial period where the clinician and patient both determine if that change led to a net benefit, side effect, or no difference in their clinical status.

SUMMARY

HTN in older adults is a common disease with different BP goal targets. Clinicians must weigh the risks and benefits of more (SBP <120–130 mm Hg) or less (SBP <150 mm Hg) intense control. Recognizing unique challenges such as multimorbidities, cognitive, pill burden, and geriatric syndromes is important in guiding clinical goals. The TTB for HTN treatment is on the order of 1 to 2 years, and so life expectancy plays another factor in determining whether to initiate, increase, or deprescribe BP medications. Some level of uncertainty will be present in these clinical decision-making but is part of geriatric care.

CLINICS CARE POINTS

• Hypertension (HTN) treatment goals in older adults require consideration of their multimorbidities, unique clinical, psychosocial and functional circumstances, overall prognosis, and goals of care.

- Deprescribing HTN medications should include a discussion with patients on its risks versus benefits, medication tapering schedules required, and close follow-up over weeks and months to determine their net effect.
- Time to benefit of HTN control helps guide clinicians on assessing polypharmacy and deprescribing decisions for older adults.

DISCLOSURE

The author has nothing to disclose.

REFERENCES

1. Whelton PK, Carey RM, Aronow WS, et al. 2017 ACC/AHA/AAPA/ABC/ACPM/AGS/APhA/ASH/ASPC/NMA/PCNA guideline for the prevention, detection, evaluation, and management of high blood pressure in adults: executive summary: a report of the American College of Cardiology/American Heart Association Task Force on Clinical Practice Guidelines. Hypertension 2018;71(6):1269–324 [Epub 2017 Nov 13. Erratum in: Hypertension. 2018 Jun;71(6):e136-e139; Erratum in: Hypertension. 2018 Sep;72(3):e33. PMID: 29133354.

2. Aubert CE, Ha JK, Kim HM, et al. Clinical outcomes of modifying hypertension treatment intensity in older adults treated to low blood pressure. J Am Geriatr Soc 2021;69(10):2831–41 [Epub 2021 Jun 7. PMID: 34097300; PMCID: PMC8497391].

3. James PA, Oparil S, Carter BL, et al. 2014 evidence-based guideline for the management of high blood pressure in adults: report from the panel members appointed to the Eighth Joint National Committee (JNC 8). JAMA 2014;311(5):507–20 [Erratum in: JAMA. 2014 May 7;311(17):1809. PMID: 24352797].

4. Qaseem A, Wilt TJ, Rich R, et al. Clinical guidelines committee of the American College of physicians and the commission on health of the public and science of the American academy of family physicians, Fitterman N, Barry MJ, Horwitch CA, Iorio A, McLean RM. Pharmacologic treatment of hypertension in adults aged 60 Years or older to higher versus lower blood pressure targets: a clinical practice guideline from the American College of physicians and the American academy of family physicians. Ann Intern Med 2017;166(6):430–7. https://doi.org/10.7326/M16-1785 [Epub 2017 Jan 17. Erratum in: Ann Intern Med. 2018 Apr 3;168(7):530-532. PMID: 28135725.)].

5. SPRINT Research Group, Wright JT Jr, Williamson JD, Whelton PK, et al. A randomized trial of intensive versus standard blood-pressure control. N Engl J Med 2015;373(22):2103–16. Nov 9.[Erratum in: N Engl J Med. 2017 Dec 21;377(25):2506. PMID: 26551272; PMCID: PMC4689591].

6. Unger T, Borghi C, Charchar F, et al. 2020 International Society of Hypertension global hypertension practice guidelines. J Hypertens 2020;38(6):982–1004. PMID: 32371787.

7. Zhang W, Zhang S, Deng Y, et al, STEP Study Group. Trial of intensive blood-pressure control in older patients with hypertension. N Engl J Med 2021;385(14):1268–79. Epub 2021 Aug 30. PMID: 34491661.).

8. Jaffe MG, Lee GA, Young JD, et al. Improved blood pressure control associated with a large-scale hypertension program. JAMA 2013;310(7):699–705.

9. Bennett A, Chow CK, Chou M, et al. Efficacy and safety of quarter-dose blood pressure-lowering agents: a systematic review and meta-analysis of randomized

controlled trials. Hypertension 2017;70(1):85–93. Epub 2017 Jun 5. PMID: 28584013.).

10. Calhoun DA, Lacourcière Y, Chiang YT, et al. Triple antihypertensive therapy with amlodipine, valsartan, and hydrochlorothiazide: a randomized clinical trial. Hypertension 2009;54(1):32–9. Epub 2009 May 26. PMID: 19470877.

11. Chrysant SG, Littlejohn T 3rd, Izzo JL Jr, et al. Triple-Combination therapy with olmesartan, amlodipine, and hydrochlorothiazide in black and non-black study participants with hypertension: the TRINITY randomized, double-blind, 12-week, parallel-group study. Am J Cardiovasc Drugs 2012;12(4):233–43.

12. Jamerson K, Weber MA, Bakris GL, et al. ACCOMPLISH Trial Investigators. Benazepril plus amlodipine or hydrochlorothiazide for hypertension in high-risk patients. N Engl J Med 2008;359(23):2417–28.

13. Salam A, Kanukula R, Atkins E, et al. Efficacy and safety of dual combination therapy of blood pressure-lowering drugs as initial treatment for hypertension: a systematic review and meta-analysis of randomized controlled trials. J Hypertens 2019;37(9):1768–74. PMID: 30986788.

14. Webster R, Salam A, de Silva HA, et al, TRIUMPH Study Group. Fixed low-dose triple combination antihypertensive medication vs usual care for blood pressure control in patients with mild to moderate hypertension in Sri Lanka: a randomized clinical trial. JAMA 2018;320(6):566–79 [Erratum in: JAMA. 2018 Nov 13;320(18): 1940. PMID: 30120478; PMCID: PMC6583010].

15. Finucane TE, Christmas C, Travis K. Tube feeding in patients with advanced dementia: a review of the evidence. JAMA 1999;282(14):1365–70.

16. Gillick MR. Rethinking the role of tube feeding in patients with advanced dementia. N Engl J Med 2000;342(3):206–10. PMID: 10639550.

17. Cai X, Campbell N, Khan B, et al. Long-term anticholinergic use and the aging brain. Alzheimers Dement 2013;9(4):377–85.

18. Lee SJ, Kim CM. Individualizing prevention for older adults. J Am Geriatr Soc 2018;66(2):229–34 [Epub 2017 Nov 20. PMID: 29155445; PMCID: PMC5809295.].

Polypharmacy in Treatment of Behavioral Issues in Dementia—Use of Atypical Antipsychotics

Jason Jalil, MD[a],*, Pargol Nazarian, PharmD[b],
Hans F. von Walter, MD[c]

KEYWORDS

- Polypharmacy • Dementia • Behavioral disturbances • Antipsychotics
- Deprescribing

KEY POINTS

- Behavioral and psychological symptoms of dementia (BPSD) presents a cohort of symptoms in dementia syndromes that pose a risk to patients and caregivers in terms of morbidity and mortality.
- Current research and literature has limited studies on effective pharmacologic and nonpharmacologic interventions for the treatment of BPSD. Although controversial, atypical antipsychotics seem to be one of the most used treatment modalities, with modest efficacy at best.
- The approach to a patient with BPSD must be judicious, as is the selection of an appropriate treatment regimen. Given the limited efficacy of any single medication, the risk and hazards of polypharmacy are elevated in this treatment demographic.
- The use of antipsychotics is warranted in specific scenarios, and in such, the risk/benefit analysis of antipsychotic use should be performed regularly, with adequate monitoring and attempts at deprescribing or gradual dose reduction.

INTRODUCTION

Among dementia syndromes, behavioral and psychological symptoms of dementia (BPSD) presents as one of the more difficult problematic markers of advancing illness.

[a] Department of Psychiatry and Biobehavioral Sciences, Semel Institute for Neuroscience and Human Behavior, University of California, 300 Medical Plaza, Suite 2200, Los Angeles, CA 90095, USA; [b] Department of Pharmacy, Stewart & Lynda Resnick Neuropsychiatric Hospital, University of California, 150 Medical Plaza, Room 4235, Los Angeles, CA 90095, USA; [c] Division of Geriatric Mental Health, Department of Psychiatry, Greater Los Angeles VA Healthcare System, 11301 Wilshire Boulevard, Building 401, Los Angeles, CA 90036, USA
* Corresponding author.
E-mail address: JJalil@mednet.ucla.edu

Clin Geriatr Med 38 (2022) 641–652
https://doi.org/10.1016/j.cger.2022.05.006
0749-0690/22/© 2022 Elsevier Inc. All rights reserved.

BPSD includes symptoms ranging from depression and anxiety to insomnia, restlessness, agitation, and frank psychosis. Up to 97% of community-dwelling patients with dementia may experience or exhibit BPSD. The presence of BPSD correlates with increased rates of hospitalization, institutionalization, caregiver burnout, morbidity, and mortality.[1] Acute onset of behavioral symptoms may occur in the presence of delirium, uncontrolled pain, a parallel medical illness, or toxidrome; insidious development, however, is often consistent with progression of the underlying neurodegenerative process. The cause of BPSD should be investigated before initiating any pharmacologic or nonpharmacologic treatment strategy. With the presence of more severe or problematic symptoms, practitioners are more likely to prescribe an antipsychotic, given the proven efficacy of reducing psychotic symptoms in patients without formal neurocognitive disorders. This practice exists despite large randomized controlled trials for BPSD or the lack of a Food and Drug Administration (FDA) approval of any medication for BPSD. The efficacy of antipsychotics in these scenarios is modest, at best, and is associated with significant risks. Despite this, antipsychotics are one of the largest classes of drugs used for these patients, and oftentimes, a subset of patients is prescribed more than one antipsychotic for the treatment of BPSD.

Specific to this topic, there is no consensus on a standardized definition for polypharmacy. We have adopted the notion that antipsychotic polypharmacy is the coprescription (or coadministration) of 2 or more antipsychotic drugs for an individual.

Polypharmacy and Dementia

The detrimental risks and effects of polypharmacy and off-label medication use in older adults are well established in literature. Community-dwelling adults with dementia generally have more prescription medications than those without dementia.[2] Increased medication regimen complexities were observed to correlate with higher rates of medication noncompliance as well as increased rates of hospitalization in the geriatric population. There is also an increased likelihood of falls and hip fractures, cognitive impairment, and functional decline.[3] In one meta-analysis of 47 studies looking into the effects of polypharmacy on mortality, every discrete medication added to a patient's medication list conferred an adjusted increased risk ratio of 1.08.[2] Dose-dependent increases in the number of medications taken are positively associated with increased risks of concurrent dementia.[2] In 2018, 13.9% of older adults with dementia were found to have concurrent prescriptions from at least 3 different central nervous system (CNS)-acting drug classes, a phenomenon referred to as "CNS-active polypharmacy."[4]

Adults with dementia are susceptible to the CNS-acting effects of several medications often implicated in polypharmacy. This may include the deliriogenic effects of anticholinergic medications (such as benzodiazepines and bladder antispasmodics) or apathy, oversedation, and akathisia from antipsychotics. Increases in the total number of prescribed medications further the risk of the prescription of "potentially inappropriate medications," as defined by American Geriatrics Society Beers Criteria.[5] In one study of older military veterans, 40% of those with polypharmacy (defined as 5 or more prescription medications) were simultaneously taking at least 1 PIM while not prescribed a potentially beneficial medication.[6] This raises a concern that polypharmacy may contribute toward worse health outcomes due to underutilization of beneficial medications.

Behavioral Disturbances of Dementia

BPSD complicates the issue of polypharmacy. BPSD is the neuropsychiatric manifestation of emotional, perceptual, or behavioral disturbances within the context of dementia. These symptoms span multiple psychological domains including, but not limited to, delusions, hallucinations, depression, apathy, agitation, physical and verbal aggression, wandering, disinhibition, and irritability. Up to 97% of community-dwelling adults with dementia have reported at least one symptom at some point during the course of their illness, most commonly depression.[1] Although the cause of BPSD is likely due to the underlying neurodegenerative process, there are both static and dynamic risk factors in the etiopathogenesis of these symptoms. Dynamic, or modifiable, factors may include pain, acute medical issues, sleep disturbances, medication adverse effects, overstimulation (or conversely, understimulation), and lack of behavioral structure.[7] Unmodifiable static factors include type of dementia and stage, neurologic issues, psychiatric history, personality, and life events.[7] BPSD can be a major clinical burden for caregivers, nursing home staff, and clinicians, resulting in an increased risk of caregiver burnout and harm to either patient or caregiver. If left untreated without intervention, BPSD may ultimately lead to acute hospital admission and need for intensive care.[8]

Treatment Strategies for Behavioral Disturbances in Dementia

Before initiating any treatments for BPSD, a thorough screening for any modifiable or treatable contributors (above) should be completed. Pharmacologic and nonpharmacological treatment strategies are both effective for the treatment of BPSD. Among guidelines for the treatment of BPSD, it is encouraged to have patients, families, and caregivers involved in treatment planning, including discussions about goals of care, and providing education on the risks and benefits of all treatment options.[9]

Nonpharmacological Treatments

There is an international consensus that nonpharmacologic approaches should be used as first-line treatment modalities.[10–13] Nonpharmacological treatments can offer similar efficacy to pharmacologic treatments without the risk of serious adverse events.[14] Among specific nonpharmacologic strategies studied for BPSD, behavioral management techniques and music therapy show the most promise.[15] Although these treatments offer a safer alternative to pharmacologic approaches, they require adequate staffing, time, and training, which may not always be feasible. These treatments should be continued concurrently if medications are initiated. A detailed assessment of underlying causes and contributing factors should be performed to aid in the development of individualized treatment plans. Caregiver education and support, as well as environmental structuring for the patient, are the cornerstones of these nonpharmacological interventions.[16]

Pharmacologic Treatments—Antipsychotics

A series of Smith, Kline & French Laboratories adverts from the 1950s hailed chlorpromazine as an answer to the need for "prompt control of senile agitation," around the time that Terman published one of the first articles on the matter titled "Treatment of senile agitation with chlorpromazine".[17] Since then, much has advanced, not just in developments in psychopharmacology, but our understanding of psychiatric illnesses and the human condition.

There is a strong consensus among many international guidelines that any pharmacologic intervention for BPSD should be reserved for severe or refractory cases.[10–13] These are circumstances where nonpharmacological approaches have failed to alleviate clinical and psychosocial distress from BPSD, or there is a risk for imminent harm to the patient or others. Currently, no medication in the United States carries an FDA-approval for the treatment of BPSD. Notably, although it lacks regulatory approval in the United States, risperidone has approval in Canada, Australia, New Zealand, and the United Kingdom for the treatment of BPSD.[18] Among the many classes of medications used off-label for this indication, antipsychotics seem to have the most evidence and continue to be the most commonly used.[19]

Current evidence supports the use of antipsychotics to target psychosis (hallucinations, delusions) and aggression only.[20] Their use to target any other symptoms would be considered inappropriate.[21] The American Psychiatric Association (APA) guidelines on use of atypical antipsychotics in BPSD stress the use of atypical antipsychotics when symptoms are severe, dangerous, and/or cause significant distress to the patient and caregiver(s).[10] Clinicians will often approach pharmacologic treatment of BPSD with prescribing algorithms that mirror similar symptoms in younger adults. Prescribed antipsychotics for BPSD have demonstrated little to modest overall benefit in high-quality clinical trials.[22]

An Agency for Healthcare Research and Quality (AHRQ) Comparative Effectiveness Review concluded that aripiprazole (for overall BPSD), olanzapine (for agitation), and risperidone (for psychosis, agitation, and overall BPSD) are effective treatment options.[20] Most of the evidence for quetiapine suggested that it is ineffective for BPSD.[20] These studies had modest effect sizes at best. The Clinical Antipsychotic Trials of Intervention Effectiveness-Alzheimer's Disease study affirmed modest efficacy in the treatment of BPSD with the aforementioned atypical antipsychotics, although with significant discontinuation of treatment due to adverse effects.[23] Additional reviews and meta-analyses echo the AHRQ results that the aforementioned antipsychotics exhibit a small but statistically significant effect size in the treatment of BPSD.[24,25]

One recent network meta-analysis found not a single atypical antipsychotic to be consistently better across all effectiveness and safety outcomes.[25] Atypical antipsychotics are generally preferred over typical antipsychotics due to their tolerability profile. Symptom improvement is usually seen within 1 to 4 weeks of antipsychotic initiation in those who respond,[26] and recent data support that the reduction in symptoms of BPSD early in the treatment (at 2 weeks) is significantly associated with subsequent treatment response at week 8.[27]

Data for the role of newer antipsychotics are scant. Promising data is emerging for pimavanserin and brexpiprazole; however, it may be too early to tell if these agents will exhibit a larger effect size or have an improved overall safety profile.[19]

Antipsychotic use in patients with dementia must be balanced against their serious adverse effect profile. Meta-analyses demonstrated a 1.5 to 1.7-fold greater risk of mortality in patients with dementia who use antipsychotics.[21] The most frequent causes of death include cardiac-related events and infection.[24] In 2005, the FDA issued a "Black Box Warning," its most stringent warning for medications, to atypical antipsychotics used in patients with dementia-related psychosis due to an increased risk of death.[28] In 2008, this warning expanded to include typical antipsychotics after data emerged suggesting that the risk of mortality is similar, if not more, with first generation antipsychotics.[29] Subsequent data has further reaffirmed the increased risk of mortality with antipsychotics,[30] and the rate of mortality seems to be highest within the first 30 to 40 days of treatment initiation. Observational data suggests that patients with prolonged antipsychotic exposure have higher rates of mortality.[31]

Antipsychotics also have potential for other well-known adverse reactions. The most serious being a 2-fold increased risk of cerebrovascular events, including stroke.[21] Other side effects include extrapyramidal symptoms (including parkinsonism), metabolic syndrome, sedation, gait abnormalities (often leading to falls), anticholinergic effects, orthostatic hypotension, and QTc prolongation.[7,24]

The use of antipsychotics may predispose a patient to the development of neuro-leptic malignant syndrome (NMS). NMS is a life-threatening idiosyncratic reaction to neuroleptic drugs characterized by fever, altered mental status, muscle rigidity, and autonomic instability.[32] Although NMS can occur with virtually all antipsychotics, the risk is greatest with high potency agents or during the initiation or increase in dose of a neuroleptic medication.[33] Not surprisingly, the use of 2 or more antipsychotics also confers a greater risk of developing NMS,[34] especially when combined with the factors above. Although age is not an independent risk factor for the development of NMS, common risk factors such as dehydration, physical exhaustion, unprotected exposure to heat, hyponatremia, iron deficiency, malnutrition, physical trauma (eg, falls), thyrotoxicosis, alcohol intoxication, psychoactive substance misuse, and the presence of a structural or functional brain disorder such as encephalitis, an intracra-nial tumor, delirium, or dementia may be more present among older adults.[33,35]

Given these serious and well-known adverse events associated with antipsychotic use, continuous evaluation of risks and benefits is crucial throughout the course of treatment, as is interval assessment for dose reduction.

Pharmacologic Treatments—Alternative Agents

There is a lack of consensus for using other therapeutic classes to treat BPSD. Selec-tive serotonin reuptake inhibitors (SSRIs), particularly citalopram, have the most robust evidence.[36] Studies on sertraline and escitalopram in BPSD continue to demonstrate promising evidence in the management of agitation in dementia without the associated cardiac risks of QTc prolongation.[37,38] Several studies suggest that SSRIs such as citalopram and sertraline are more effective than placebo or just as effective as antipsychotics for agitation and irritability. Symptom improvement can be seen in 2 to 3 weeks with these agents and tolerability is often greater than antipsy-chotics.[26] However, SSRIs have the potential for their own severe adverse effects including QTc prolongation (particularly with citalopram) and hyponatremia.[7] An inter-national Delphi consensus study on BPSD management prioritized citalopram and treatment of pain with analgesics above antipsychotics for the overall treatment of BPSD and agitation.[39]

Current literature does not support the primary use of other psychotropic medica-tion classes such as benzodiazepines, stimulants, typical (first generation) antipsy-chotics, and long-acting injectable antipsychotics in BPSD. Anticonvulsants are generally discouraged due to the lack of efficacy, such as valproate, or poor tolera-bility and drug–drug interactions, as seen with carbamazepine.[26] There are limited data to support the use of acetylcholinesterase inhibitors for severe behavioral symp-toms, especially in individuals with dementia due to AD, vascular disease, and Lewy Body disease. Acetylcholinesterase inhibitors, such as donepezil, may be more effec-tive for depression, dysphoria, apathy, and anxiety symptoms than for agitation or aggression.[7] Memantine can be beneficial for agitation, aggression, and delusions. The benefit of these agents is sometimes delayed up to 3 to 6 months, thus there is lower utility in acute treatment of BPSD.[26]

The most common type of polypharmacy in patients at least 5 years after a diag-nosis of Alzheimer dementia was an antipsychotic plus an antidepressant, with a prev-alence of at least 8% in a large-scale European review.[40] Concerningly, that review also demonstrated a prevalence of at least 2% and 1%, respectively, of patients on 2 or more antipsychotics or antidepressants during this same time interval. Despite this, the APA has not released practice guidelines on the use of antidepressants in combination with antipsychotics in the treatment of BPSD and recommends judicious patient-centered clinical judgment when considering their use.

Antipsychotic Polypharmacy

There are identified short-term and long-term scenarios where antipsychotic polypharmacy is evidenced, or even warranted. Oftentimes, short-term polypharmacy occurs in an acute setting, where a rapid response is desired and medical management of patients is feasible. One example includes a patient prescribed one particular antipsychotic is given an "as needed" or PRN (lit: *pro re nata*) dose of a second antipsychotic that might only be available in a formulation suitable for emergent agitation (such as an oral dissolvable tablet, an intravenous or intramuscular formulation). Another example would be during a cross-titration to monotherapy, where 2 antipsychotics are concurrently prescribed with the goal to taper one medication to discontinuation while titrating the dose of the second. Long-term antipsychotic polypharmacy in dementia is more controversial and currently there are no data to support its practice. In long-term use, although not recommended, antipsychotic polypharmacy may be justified if the patient is on clozapine augmented with a second antipsychotic or if a patient with continued behavioral disturbances has 3 or more failed trials of antipsychotic monotherapy, including clozapine. One clinical scenario to consider is a comorbid diagnosis of dementia alongside a previously existing primary affective or psychotic disorder. In such a case, a patient may be on a longstanding antipsychotic indicated for the primary psychotic disorder. If they were to develop dementia with behavioral disturbances, a second antipsychotic may potentially be added to target BPSD, especially if they are unable to tolerate higher doses or switch their initial antipsychotic.

If 2 antipsychotics are warranted, it is recommended to avoid the use of 2 high potency agents. Additionally, to achieve maximal efficacy, it is prudent to avoid the use of 2 agents that have similar dopamine-2 affinity, such as clozapine and quetiapine.

Deprescribing Antipsychotics

Psychosis in individuals with dementia shows a low prevalence. This combined with modest efficacy and potential for significant harm, provides a worthwhile opportunity for deprescribing.

Deprescribing is "the planned and supervised process of dose reduction or stopping of medication that might be causing harm, or no longer be of benefit."[21] The APA recommends stopping antipsychotics after 4 weeks if there is no clinically significant response.[10] Furthermore, they recommend attempting to taper off an antipsychotic within 4 months of initiation in patients who show adequate response to antipsychotics.

A 2018 Cochrane review concluded that antipsychotics can be successfully discontinued in individuals with dementia without exacerbating their behavior.[41] They found benefits especially for those with milder symptoms, however, clarified that those with more severe symptoms may benefit from continuing treatment. Other trials have also investigated withdrawal of antipsychotics and reached a similar conclusion that antipsychotics can be successfully removed for most patients with BPSD.[42,43]

A Canadian workgroup initiated the Deprescribing Guidelines in the Elderly Project.[44] Their aim was to provide evidence-based recommendations and tools for clinicians for deprescribing. This workgroup has a specific algorithm for antipsychotics for BPSD and insomnia (**Fig. 1**). They predict successful antipsychotic cessation occurs in individuals who require a lower dose for symptom control and have lower severity of symptoms at baseline.[21] Not all individuals will be able to stop antipsychotics successfully. Guidance on treatment options when BPSD reappears is also provided in the algorithm.

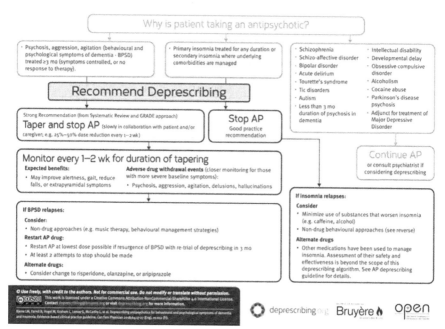

Fig. 1. Antipsychotic deprescribing algorithm. (*From* Bjerre LM, Farrell B, Hogel M, et al. Deprescribing antipsychotics for behavioural and psychological symptoms of dementia and insomnia: Evidence-based clinical practice guideline. Can Fam Physician. 2018;64(1):17-27; with permission.)

Although the importance of deprescribing and individuals who would benefit from it have been extensively delineated, relatively little information is available to guide appropriate dose reduction of individual agents. An increase in BPSD after abrupt discontinuation of an antipsychotic may reflect an adverse drug withdrawal event rather than a return of symptoms. As such, antipsychotics should be gradually tapered off over time and not abruptly discontinued when clinically feasible.[31] Several

Table 1
Tapering schedule for individual antipsychotics

Antipsychotic	Time Between Gradual Dose Reduction	Estimated Time to Discontinuation
Aripiprazole (Abilify)	2 mo	4 mo
Olanzapine (Zyprexa)	2–4 wk	4–8 wk
Quetiapine (Seroquel)	2 wk	4 wk
Risperidone (Risperdal)	2–3 wk	4–6 wk

Data from Tjia J, Reidenberg MM, Hunnicutt JN, et al. Approaches to Gradual Dose Reduction of Chronic Off-Label Antipsychotics Used for Behavioral and Psychological Symptoms of Dementia. Consult Pharm. 2015;30(10):599-611. https://doi.org/10.4140/TCP.n.2015.599.

resources provide broad recommendations of reducing the dose of an antipsychotic by 50% every 2 weeks until discontinuation.[21,45] Tjia and colleagues used pharmacokinetic principles and empiric data to develop a theoretically based protocol for gradual dose reduction of individual antipsychotics (**Table 1**).[31] The ultimate decision to taper the antipsychotic versus abrupt discontinuation and the tapering schedule will depend on the severity of the BPSD symptoms at baseline, the duration of antipsychotic use, and the potential risk of exposure compared with the potential benefit of discontinuation.

As with the initiation of an antipsychotic, careful monitoring of symptoms is required during, and after, antipsychotic deprescribing regimens are started. Objective measurements via validated rating scales, such as the Neuropsychiatric Inventory can be helpful for ongoing monitoring. Short-term monitoring includes antipsychotic withdrawal symptoms, and long-term monitoring includes reemergence of BPSD.

SUMMARY

BPSD is a frequently occurring subset of symptoms present in all dementia syndromes. The presence of symptoms such as agitation, aggression, psychosis, and insomnia often lead to higher rates of institutional-placement, hospitalization, and caregiver burnout along with increased risks of morbidity and mortality. Despite the prevalence of such conditions and the detrimental impact on patients and their families, or the health-care system and society as a whole, there exist few options for the treatment of BPSD, none of which carries an FDA-approval. Treatment options are often off-label approaches that lend to the risk of polypharmacy and potentially inappropriate medication prescribing. One such approach, the use of antipsychotics for the treatment of BPSD, has been studied extensively, although high-quality randomized control trials have been limited. Even with the data available, the effects of antipsychotics in this case are moderate at best. In light of this information, antipsychotic drugs seem to confer the best efficacy in the treatment of severe or refractory behavioral symptoms in dementia patients. Although polypharmacy with antipsychotics can be troublesome due to drug–drug interactions, unwanted side effects, the potential for permanent disability and even death, there are some clinical scenarios that may warrant the use of 2 or more antipsychotics in a patient with BPSD. As such, the use of said medications should judiciously be monitored, with an attempt to reduce the dose intervals once symptoms have resolved, or, within a short timeframe if they have proven to be ineffective. There is much in the way of the future of the treatment of these symptoms, including a greater understanding and evaluation of novel agents and more effective treatments of the behavioral problems associated with dementia.

CLINICS CARE POINTS

- Polypharmacy in the geriatric population is associated with an increased risk of dementia, and a subsequent risk of behavioral and psychological symptoms of dementia (BPSD).
- BPSD affects a significant number of patients with dementia, with depression, agitation, and insomnia as common manifestations. Without intervention, these symptoms can lead to worsened health outcomes.
- A lack of robust evidence-based pharmacologic interventions for BPSD can lead to inappropriate polypharmacy and a potential worsening of the syndrome.

- Nonpharmacologic treatments are considered first line for the treatment of BPSD. Antipsychotics should only be initiated if target symptoms are severe and pose imminent harm to the individual or others.
- Antipsychotics are modestly effective for treating aggression, agitation, and psychosis in individuals with dementia.
- Antipsychotics for BPSD should be used at the lowest effective dose for the shortest duration due to their association with severe adverse events such as death and cerebrovascular events.
- The use of 2 or more antipsychotics in the treatment of BPSD is rarely justified but specific clinical scenarios exist where its use is warranted, with appropriate monitoring.
- The risk–benefit analysis of antipsychotic use should be performed regularly.
- In individuals receiving antipsychotics for BPSD, medications can be successfully tapered off without a return of symptoms; thus, a trial of deprescribing should be attempted in most patients.

DISCLOSURE

The authors have nothing to disclose.

REFERENCES

1. Cloak N, Al Khalili Y. Behavioral and psychological symptoms in dementia. In: StatPearls [Internet]. Treasure Island (FL): StatPearls Publishing; 2022. Accessed December 20, 2021.
2. Leelakanok N, Holcombe AL, Lund BC, et al. Association between polypharmacy and death: a systematic review and meta-analysis. J Am Pharm Assoc (2003) 2017;57(6):729–38.e10.
3. Lai SW, Liao KF, Liao CC, et al. Polypharmacy correlates with increased risk for hip fracture in the elderly: a population-based study. Medicine (Baltimore) 2010;89(5):295–9.
4. Maust DT, Strominger J, Kim HM, et al. Prevalence of central nervous system-active polypharmacy among older adults with dementia in the US. JAMA 2021; 325(10):952–61.
5. Lau DT, Mercaldo ND, Harris AT, et al. Polypharmacy and potentially inappropriate medication use among community-dwelling elders with dementia. Alzheimer Dis Assoc Disord 2010;24(1):56–63.
6. Fried TR, O'Leary J, Towle V, et al. Health outcomes associated with polypharmacy in community-dwelling older adults: a systematic review. J Am Geriatr Soc 2014;62(12):2261–72.
7. Tible OP, Riese F, Savaskan E, et al. Best practice in the management of behavioural and psychological symptoms of dementia. Ther Adv Neurol Disord 2017; 10(8):297–309.
8. Thompson Coon J, Abbott R, Rogers M, et al. Interventions to reduce inappropriate prescribing of antipsychotic medications in people with dementia resident in care homes: a systematic review. J Am Med Dir Assoc 2014;15(10):706–18.
9. Ngo J, Holroyd-Leduc JM. Systematic review of recent dementia practice guidelines. Age Ageing 2015;44(1):25–33.
10. Reus VI, Fochtmann LJ, Eyler AE, et al. The American psychiatric association practice guideline on the use of antipsychotics to treat agitation or psychosis in patients with dementia. Am J Psychiatry 2016;173(5):543–6.

11. National Institute for Health and Care Excellence (NICE). Dementia: assessment, management and support for people living with dementia and their carers. Available at: https://www.nice.org.uk/guidance/ng97. Accessed January 14, 2021.
12. Moore A, Patterson C, Lee L, et al. Canadian consensus conference on the diagnosis and treatment of dementia. fourth canadian consensus conference on the diagnosis and treatment of dementia: recommendations for family physicians. Can Fam Physician 2014;60(5):433–8.
13. Laver K, Cumming RG, Dyer SM, et al. Clinical practice guidelines for dementia in Australia. Med J Aust 2016;204(5):191–3.
14. Harrison SL, Cations M, Jessop T, et al. Approaches to deprescribing psychotropic medications for changed behaviours in long-term care residents living with dementia. Drugs Aging 2019;36(2):125–36.
15. Tampi RR, Tampi DJ, Rogers K, et al. Antipsychotics in the management of behavioral and psychological symptoms of dementia: maximizing gain and minimizing harm. Neurodegener Dis Manag 2020;10(1):5–8.
16. Bessey LJ, Walaszek A. Management of behavioral and psychological symptoms of dementia. Curr Psychiatry Rep 2019;21(8):66. Published 2019 Jul 1.
17. Terman LA. Treatment of senile agitation with chlorpromazine. Geriatrics 1955; 10(11):520–2.
18. Yunusa I, El Helou ML. The use of risperidone in behavioral and psychological symptoms of dementia: a review of pharmacology, clinical evidence, regulatory approvals, and off-label use. Front Pharmacol 2020;11:596. Published 2020 May 20.
19. Caraci F, Santagati M, Caruso G, et al. New antipsychotic drugs for the treatment of agitation and psychosis in Alzheimer's disease: focus on brexpiprazole and pimavanserin. F1000Res 2020;9:F1000. https://doi.org/10.12688/f1000research. 22662.1. Faculty Rev-686.
20. Maglione M, Ruelaz Maher A, Hu J, et al. Off-label use of atypical antipsychotics: an update. Comparative Effectiveness Review No. 43. (Prepared by the Southern California Evidence-based Practice Center under Contract No. HHSA290-2007-10062- 1.). Rockville, MD: Agency for Healthcare Research and Quality; 2011. Available at: www.effectivehealthcare.ahrq.gov/reports/final.cfm.
21. Bjerre LM, Farrell B, Hogel M, et al. Deprescribing antipsychotics for behavioural and psychological symptoms of dementia and insomnia: evidence-based clinical practice guideline. Can Fam Physician 2018;64(1):17–27.
22. Ravona-Springer R, Davidson M. Considerations in psychotropic treatments in dementia–can polypharmacy be avoided? Int J Neuropsychopharmacol 2014; 17(7):1107–17.
23. Schneider LS, Tariot PN, Dagerman KS, et al. Effectiveness of atypical antipsychotic drugs in patients with Alzheimer's disease. N Engl J Med 2006;355(15): 1525–38.
24. Tampi RR, Tampi DJ, Balachandran S, et al. Antipsychotic use in dementia: a systematic review of benefits and risks from meta-analyses. Ther Adv Chronic Dis 2016;7(5):229–45.
25. Yunusa I, Alsumali A, Garba AE, et al. Assessment of reported comparative effectiveness and safety of atypical antipsychotics in the treatment of behavioral and psychological symptoms of dementia: a network meta-analysis. JAMA Netw Open 2019;2(3):e190828. Published 2019 Mar 1.
26. Mathys M. Pharmacologic management of behavioral and psychological symptoms of major neurocognitive disorder. Ment Health Clin 2018;8(6):284–93. Published 2018 Nov 1.

27. Nagata T, Shinagawa S, Yoshida K, et al. Early improvements of individual symptoms with antipsychotics predict subsequent treatment response of neuropsychiatric symptoms in alzheimer's disease: a re-analysis of the CATIE-AD study. J Clin Psychiatry 2020;81(2):19m12961. Published 2020 Feb 11.
28. US Food and Drug Administration. Public health advisory: deaths with antipsychotics in elderly patients with behavioral disturbances. Available at: https://wayback.archive-it.org/7993/20170113112252/http://www.fda.gov/Drugs/DrugSafety/PostmarketDrugSafetyInformationforPatientsandProviders/ucm053171.htm. Accessed December 10, 2021.
29. US Food and Drug Administration. Information for healthcare professionals: conventional antipsychotics. Available at: https://wayback.archive-it.org/7993/20170722190727/https://www.fda.gov/Drugs/DrugSafety/PostmarketDrugSafetyInformationforPatientsandProviders/ucm124830.htm. Accessed December 10, 2021.
30. Ballard C, Hanney ML, Theodoulou M, et al. The dementia antipsychotic withdrawal trial (DART-AD): long-term follow-up of a randomised placebo-controlled trial. Lancet Neurol 2009;8(2):151–7.
31. Tjia J, Reidenberg MM, Hunnicutt JN, et al. Approaches to gradual dose reduction of chronic off-label antipsychotics used for behavioral and psychological symptoms of dementia. Consult Pharm 2015;30(10):599–611.
32. Berman BD. Neuroleptic malignant syndrome: a review for neurohospitalists. Neurohospitalist 2011;1(1):41–7.
33. Berardi D, Amore M, Keck PE, et al. Clinical and pharmacological risk factors for neuroleptic malignant syndrome : a case control study. Biol Psychiatry 1998;44:748–54.
34. Bhanushali MJ, Tuite PJ. The evaluation and management of patients with neuroleptic malignant syndrome. Neurol Clin 2004;22(2):389–411.
35. Keck PE, Pope HG, Cohen BM, et al. Risk factors for neuroleptic malignant syndrome: a case-control study. Arch Gen Psychiatry 1989;46(10):914–8.
36. Porsteinsson AP, Drye LT, Pollock BG, et al. Effect of citalopram on agitation in Alzheimer disease: the CitAD randomized clinical trial. JAMA 2014;311(7):682–91.
37. Ho T, Pollock BG, Mulsant BH, et al. R- and S-citalopram concentrations have differential effects on neuropsychiatric scores in elders with dementia and agitation. Br J Clin Pharmacol 2016;82(3):784–92.
38. Farina N, Morrell L, Banerjee S. What is the therapeutic value of antidepressants in dementia? A narrative review. Int J Geriatr Psychiatry 2017;32(1):32–49.
39. Kales HC, Lyketsos CG, Miller EM, et al. Management of behavioral and psychological symptoms in people with Alzheimer's disease: an international Delphi consensus. Int Psychogeriatr 2019;31(1):83–90.
40. Orsel K, Taipale H, Tolppanen AM, et al. Psychotropic drugs use and psychotropic polypharmacy among persons with Alzheimer's disease. Eur Neuropsychopharmacol 2018;28(11):1260–9.
41. Van Leeuwen E, Petrovic M, van Driel ML, et al. Withdrawal versus continuation of long-term antipsychotic drug use for behavioural and psychological symptoms in older people with dementia [published online ahead of print, 2018 Mar 30]. Cochrane Database Syst Rev 2018;3(3):CD007726.
42. Ruths S, Straand J, Nygaard HA, et al. Stopping antipsychotic drug therapy in demented nursing home patients: a randomized, placebo-controlled study–the Bergen District Nursing Home Study (BEDNURS). Int J Geriatr Psychiatry 2008;23(9):889–95.

43. Brodaty H, Aerts L, Harrison F, et al. Antipsychotic deprescription for older adults in long-term care: the HALT study. J Am Med Dir Assoc 2018;19(7):592–600.e7.
44. Deprescribing.org. Available at: https://www.deprescribing.org. Accessed January 15, 2022.
45. Bravo-José P, Sáez-Lleó CI, Peris-Martí JF. Deprescribing antipsychotics in long term care patients with dementia. Deprescribing antipsychotics in long term care patients with dementia. Farm Hosp 2019;43(4):140–5. Published 2019 Jul 1.

Polypharmacy in Nursing Homes

Elaine Roh, MD[a], Esteban Cota, MD[b], Jason P. Lee, MD[b], Ruth Madievsky, PharmD[c], Manuel A. Eskildsen, MD, MPH[a],*

KEYWORDS

- Nursing home • Frail • Potentially inappropriate medications
- Adverse drug events/reactions • Drug–drug interactions • Deprescribing

KEY POINTS

- Older adults in the nursing home tend to be frailer than community-dwelling older adults.
- Most frequently prescribed medications in nursing homes in the United States are gastrointestinal, psychotropic, and pain medications.
- Detailed review of medications should be done on admission to the nursing home and when the patient presents a new symptom or concern that may be an adverse reaction from one or more medications.
- Deprescribing can be achieved using tools to identify inappropriate medications and tapering or stopping medications with close monitoring.

INTRODUCTION

As the geriatric population is expected to grow, the number of individuals in nursing homes, whether for short-term rehabilitation or long-term custodial care, will also increase. Currently, approximately 14% of the US population is aged 65 years and older. This group makes up 33% of prescription drug purchases, and this number is anticipated to grow to 50% by the year 2050.[1] Polypharmacy is the use of many medications and the number for the cut off can vary, based on the purposes of research and clinical setting. Older adults have more medical conditions and thus require more medications. Polypharmacy can be appropriate or problematic. When appropriate, medications are prescribed based on best evidence with the goal of improving quality of life and longevity while reducing harm. When inappropriate or problematic, medications are prescribed not

a Department of Internal Medicine, Division of Geriatrics, University of California, 10945 Le Conte Avenue, Suite 2339, Los Angeles, CA 90095, USA; b Department of Geriatric Psychiatry, University of California, 760 Westwood Plaza, Los Angeles, CA 90095, USA; c Division of General Internal Medicine & Health Services Research, University of California, 1100 Glendon Avenue, Suite 850, Los Angeles, CA 90024, USA
* Corresponding author.
E-mail address: meskildsen@mednet.ucla.edu

Clin Geriatr Med 38 (2022) 653–666
https://doi.org/10.1016/j.cger.2022.05.007
0749-0690/22/© 2022 Elsevier Inc. All rights reserved.

geriatric.theclinics.com

Abbreviations	
COX	Cyclooxygenase
H2	Histamine H2-receptor antagonists
CNS	central nervous system
GI	gastrointestinal
AGS	American Geriatrics Society

based on evidence and risks outweigh the benefits.[2,3] The concern in polypharmacy is derived from its possible complications, which will be further discussed in this article.

NURSING HOMES IN THE UNITED STATES

In the United States, common reasons for admission to nursing homes include impairment in activities of daily living (ADLs), need for assistance from licensed individuals, and cognitive impairment with associated behavioral syndromes.[4] Nursing home patients are frailer and more vulnerable compared with community-dwelling older adults. Individuals residing in nursing homes also have multiple chronic conditions and a higher incidence of functional and cognitive impairment.[5]

Based on 2016 Centers for Disease Control and Prevention data, individuals in nursing homes can be separated by short-term stay of less than 100 days or long-term stay of 100 days and greater. Long-term residents of nursing homes are expected to be frailer, have more chronic conditions, and be prescribed more medications. Patients in both groups have similar percentages of common comorbid conditions:

- Depression: 42.6% in short stay versus 53% in long stay
- Diabetes: 37% in short stay versus 32.2% in long stay
- Hypertension: 76.8% in short stay versus 75.8% in long stay

The prescription pattern and polypharmacy can be thought to be similar among short- and long-term nursing home residents. One difference noted was in Alzheimer's or other dementia syndromes, which made up 36.7% for those in short stay compared with 58.9% in long stay. Overall, among the long-term care provided in nursing homes, adult day service centers, home health agencies, hospice, and resident care communities, nursing homes had the highest prevalence of Alzheimer's disease.[6]

CONCERN OF POLYPHARMACY IN NURSING HOMES

As the body ages, there are physiologic changes that affect the ability to absorb, distribute, metabolize, and excrete medications.[7] Owing to decreased strength, endurance, and reduced physiologic functioning, nursing home residents are more likely to have difficulty with metabolizing medications.[8]

In the 2004 National Nursing Home survey, 40% of nursing home residents were on nine or more medications, increased from 32% in the 1996 survey. Polypharmacy was associated with white race, presence of several comorbidities, and age 85 years and less. It is thought that nursing home residents older than 85 may have a lower number of medications as providers understand that too many medications put older adults at risk. Young nursing home patients tend to be present for acute rehab and recovery, thus receive more medications.[7]

Most frequently prescribed medications, hence associated with polypharmacy, in nursing homes in the United States include:

- Gastrointestinal medications: 47.5% laxatives, 43.3% acid/peptic disorder medications
- Psychiatric medications: 46.3% antidepressants, 25.9% antipsychotics or antimanics
- Pain relievers: 46.3% nonnarcotic analgesics, 41.2% antipyretics, and 31.2% antiarthritics
- Other medications: 35% diuretics, 31.2% replenishers/regulators of electrolytes/water balance, and 23.6% angiotensin-converting enzyme inhibitors.[7]

With polypharmacy, there are increased risks of potentially inappropriate medications (PIMs), adverse drug reactions (ADRs), dangerous drug–drug and drug-disease interactions, poor adherence, and prescribing cascades. Polypharmacy is also associated with increased costs. Aside from the cost of medications, more medications require more time for staff to prepare and administer. There are also higher costs in managing complications associated with medication adverse or side effects. In addition, polypharmacy has been linked to decreased cognitive function and dementia, including more rapid cognitive decline in the setting of medications with psychotropic or anticholinergic side effects. A population-based study showed that a long duration of polypharmacy is associated with higher risk of acute renal failure. Although polypharmacy is associated with increased hospitalizations, it has not been consistently associated with increased falls, fractures, and mortality.[3,9]

Frail nursing home residents, particularly those diagnosed with dementia, are not only more likely to be started on PIMs but also less likely to have them discontinued. PIMs are medications that have risks that outweigh benefits. One survey showed that 40% of nursing home residents have an order for at least one PIM.[1,10] When analyzing outcomes of polypharmacy, considering PIMs may be more important than the number of medications.[3]

EVALUATION OF POLYPHARMACY IN THE NURSING HOME

When addressing polypharmacy, medication prescribing or deprescribing can be done efficiently by categorizing patients in groups based on frailty, fall risk, cognitive impairment, and cardiovascular comorbidities. When there are new symptoms or concerns, providers should always consider the possibility of medication-induced effects.[1] Most importantly, the provider needs to perform careful medication reconciliation. A process for medication reconciliation is:

1. Verification
2. Clarification
3. Reconciliation

Although the process can be time-consuming, creating a complete and accurate list of medications with the medication name, dosage, formulation, frequency, timing, route of administration, and indication is important. This list and medication reconciliation should be done at any transition point, including admission into, transfer between, and discharge from nursing homes.[5,11] With changing guidelines, providers should keep and remove medications as appropriate for the individual patient at the current time.[12]

Based on a systematic review and expert consensus study, the appropriateness of medication can be evaluated by the following:

1. Adherence
2. Adverse effects

3. Alternatives, such as non-pharmacological measures
4. Clinical response
5. Clinically significant drug–drug interactions
6. Complexity of medication regimen
7. Compliance with clinical practice guidelines
8. Adequate instructions
9. Contraindications[5]

Interventions targeting decreased ADRs in older adults have been successful. A recent systematic review found a 35% risk reduction in pharmacist-led interventions to decreased ADRs. Computerized decision support systems for optimization of medications are becoming more prevalent and increasing in sophistication. These systems decrease the risk of PIMs as there is integration of various patient-specific data such as kidney function or creatinine clearance and common drug–drug interactions.[9]

There are also evidence-based tools to help identify inappropriate medications, with the most common being the Beers Criteria and the Screening Tool of Older Person's Prescriptions (STOPP) and the Screening Tools to Alert Doctors to Right Treatment (START). The Beers Criteria for PIM use in older adults from the American Geriatrics Society is meant for use in individuals 65 years and older in ambulatory, acute, and institutionalized settings of care. The most recent version from 2019 has information on medications to avoid in older adults based on 30 criteria, 40 medications or classes that should be used with caution or avoided in certain medical diseases based on 16 criteria, general drug–drug interactions that should be avoided, and medications that should be avoided or dose adjusted based on kidney function.[13] Validated and evidence-based lists of inappropriate prescribing from Europe are the STOPP/START criteria. STOPP has 80 criteria for potentially inappropriate prescribing and START has 34 criteria for prescribing medications of common diseases in community-dwelling older adults.[14] In a trial carried out in the nursing home setting, patients whose medications were adjusted according to the STOPP/START criteria received significantly fewer numbers of drugs, experienced less frequent falls, and had lower medication costs.[15]

The creators of the STOPP/START criteria have also noted that the criteria can be applied in nursing homes but may have limits given shorter life expectancy in residents. A two-stage expert panel process evaluated the STOPP/START criteria and identified 22 measures of the STOPP criteria and 2 measures of the START criteria for US nursing homes.[14]

Potentially missed prescriptions from the START criteria are vaccines, including pneumococcal vaccine and seasonal influenza vaccine,[14] and PIMs from the STOPP criteria are as follows:

- Non-steroidal anti-inflammatory drugs (NSAIDs):
  - NSAIDs with anticoagulant or antiplatelet, but without proton-pump inhibitors (PPIs) prophylaxis
  - Cyclooxygenase-2 (COX-2) selective NSAIDs with cardiovascular disease
  - NSAIDs and COX-2 selective NSAIDs in setting of peptic ulcer disease without PPI or Histamine H2-receptor antagonists
- Medications affecting the central nervous system (CNS):
  - Anticholinergics or antimuscarinics with delirium or dementia
  - Antipsychotics, except quetiapine or clozapine, with Parkinsonism or Lewy body disease
  - Phenothiazines, tricyclic antidepressants, or first-generation antipsychotics
  - Benzodiazepines for longer than 4 weeks

- o Two or more drugs with antimuscarinic or anticholinergic properties
- o Two medications within the classes of hypnotics/sedatives, antidepressants, or anxiolytics
- Diabetic medications: sulfonylureas
- Medications affecting the gastrointestinal system:
  - o Oral elemental iron dose of more than 200 mg daily
  - o Prochlorperazine or metoclopramide with Parkinsonism
  - o PPI for uncomplicated peptic ulcer disease or erosive peptic esophagitis at therapeutic dosage for more than 8 weeks
- Medications affecting the kidneys:
  - o Digoxin greater than 125 mcg per day
  - o Metformin in end-stage renal disease or dialysis
  - o NSAIDs with renal failure, end-stage renal disease, or dialysis
- Medications affecting the urogenital system:
  - o Antimuscarinic drugs in dementia, cognitive impairment, glaucoma/cataracts/macular degeneration, or enlarged prostate
  - o Selective alpha-1 blockers with orthostatic hypotension
- Medications affecting the respiratory system:
  - o Systemic corticosteroids more than 14 days rather than inhaled corticosteroids for maintenance therapy
  - o Systemic corticosteroids not indicated in chronic obstructive pulmonary disease[14]

DEPRESCRIBING IN THE NURSING HOME

After a review and evaluation of medications, the next step in addressing polypharmacy is deprescribing. Deprescribing is the process of tapering or stopping drugs to minimize polypharmacy and improving patient outcomes.[16]

General Steps in Deprescribing:

1. Identify PIMs
2. Determine if the medication dosage can be reduced or medication stopped
3. Plan tapering
4. Monitor for withdrawal symptoms
5. Document and monitor outcomes

For deprescribing algorithms, the College of Family Physicians of Canada has evidence-based clinical practice guidelines for the deprescribing process of PPIs, antihyperglycemics, antipsychotics for behavioral and psychological symptoms of dementia and insomnia, and benzodiazepine receptor agonists (BZRAs). The University of Sydney has an evidence-based clinical practice guideline for the deprescribing process of acetylcholinesterase inhibitors (AChEIs) and memantine. There are steps that medical providers can follow including when to consider deprescribing, timeline of tapering, symptoms to monitor during or after deprescribing, and how withdrawal symptoms can be addressed.[17]

With a team-based approach and ongoing monitoring, the likelihood of successful reductions in polypharmacy without the reintroduction of agents will increase.[18] A meta-analysis of deprescribing in the nursing home population showed a significantly reduced number of residents with PIMs by 59%. In a subgroup analysis, medication review-directed deprescribing interventions reduced all-cause mortality by 26% and reduction in the number of falls by 24%.[19] Overall, medical providers should also take into consideration remaining life expectancy, time until benefit, goals of care, and treatment targets. With nursing home patients varying from acute rehabilitation to long-term care, patients who are preparing to return to the community, and those who may need hospice care, each patient needs a tailored approach.[20]

POLYPHARMACY AND KEY MEDICATIONS USED IN THE NURSING HOME
Psychotropic Medications

There is a high rate of utilization of psychotropic medications in nursing homes, which is a concern due to the potential for serious adverse or side effects. Maust and colleagues analyzed data from the Aging, Demographics, and Memory Study and found 41.4% of participants who were over 70 years old with dementia and were taking a psychotropic medication. Moreover, 84% of those taking a psychotropic medication were nursing home residents compared with 28.6% who were community dwellers.[21]

Depressive symptoms are common among nursing home residents, with documented rates as high as 35%. Antidepressant prescribing in the United States increased from 21.9% in 1996 to 47.5% in 2006. Findings from this study suggest that the increase in use of antidepressants is associated with increased time in a facility, the co-prescribing of a sedative/hypnotic medication, and more time spent with nurses and nurse aides. Factors associated with a decrease in antidepressants include the greater presence of physicians and medical directors, and the prescribing of antipsychotic and antianxiety medications.[22,23] In a Belgian study of 1730 residents from 76 different nursing homes, approximately 39.5% of residents were taking an antidepressant, most often a selective serotonin reuptake inhibitor. Bourgeois and colleagues found that some patients may be taking antidepressants for reasons other than depression, such as insomnia, anxiety, and neuropathic pain.[24]

The use of BZRAs, including benzodiazepine and z-drugs, in nursing homes deserves special attention as these medications are known to cause psychomotor and cognitive adverse effects in older adults. Concerning risks of these medications include sedation, dizziness, falls and fractures, cognitive deterioration, and delirium.[25] In a post hoc analysis, Rijksen and colleagues assessed the prevalence and appropriateness of patients taking BZRAs in 24 Dutch long-term facilities. Of 1111 residents, 64.7% used one or more psychotropic medications and 39.2% used a BZRA. The continuous use of BZRAs occurred in 22.9% of residents, and 16.3% were prescribed as needed. Appropriate indication for continuous anxiolytic BZRAs was found in only 19% of residents and for hypnotic BZRAs in 44.8% of residents. Agitation and aggression were diagnoses for 75.7% of inappropriate use of continuous anxiolytic BZRAs. Nighttime agitation accounted for 40.3% of inappropriate use of hypnotic BZRAs. All prescriptions for anxiolytic BZRAs and 81.4% of hypnotic BZRAs exceeded the recommended 4-week course.[26]

Antipsychotic medications (APMs) are commonly prescribed in nursing homes for agitation or other behavioral disturbances. Chiu and colleagues found that over one in four US nursing home residents were taking an APM at any given time, with 86% to 95% having off-label indications. The risks of APMs were profound, with an increased risk of hospitalization for infection, somnolence, urinary incontinence, and convulsions. Olanzapine was shown to quadruple the risk of hip fracture. The Food and Drug Administration has a black box warning of increased risk of mortality for APMs in patients with dementia. However, the risk of mortality increases in all patients taking APMs, regardless of the diagnosis of dementia.[27]

Deprescribing psychotropic medications, especially in patients with behavioral disturbances, can be challenging. Reasons include insufficient time to adequately review patients' medications and expressed concerns that staff were not sufficiently trained to address behavioral disturbances of patients with dementia.[28]

Anticholinergic Medications

Anticholinergics are commonly prescribed to older patients for the treatment of a variety of conditions such as urinary incontinence, irritable bowel syndrome, and Parkinson's disease.[29] The significant risks in older adults include functional and cognitive decline, falls, and institutionalization. Owing to anticholinergic effects on the central nervous system, there is a risk of cognitive impairment and acceleration of neurodegenerative processes. Cognitive decline has been observed clinically with cognitive testing and neuroimaging after use of anticholinergic medications. Owing to the anticholinergic effect on the peripheral nervous system, additional common adverse effects include dry mouth, urinary retention, constipation, paralytic ileus, tachycardia, and blurred vision.[30]

CNS medications with a high anticholinergic burden:
- Tricyclic antidepressants: amitriptyline, clomipramine, desipramine, imipramine
- Antipsychotics: chlorpromazine, clozapine, olanzapine
- Antiepileptics: carbamazepine, oxcarbazepine
- Antiparkinson medications: benztropine, trihexyphenidyl

CNS medications with a low-to-moderate anticholinergic burden:
- Antidepressants: fluoxetine, fluvoxamine, mirtazapine, nortriptyline, paroxetine, sertraline, trazodone
- Antipsychotics: haloperidol, quetiapine, ziprasidone
- Benzodiazepines
- Antiparkinson medications: amantadine, bromocriptine, carbidopa–levodopa, pramipexole, selegiline
- Opioids: codeine, fentanyl, morphine, tramadol

Common non-CNS medications with anticholinergic effects:
- Antihistamines: diphenhydramine, hydroxyzine, loratadine
- Antispasmodics: loperamide
- H2 blockers: cimetidine, ranitidine
- Bronchodilators: fluticasone-salmeterol
- Cardiovascular: digoxin, diltiazem, warfarin
- Corticosteroids: cortisone, dexamethasone, methylprednisolone, prednisone
- Diuretics: chlorthalidone, furosemide
- Overactive bladder medications: oxybutynin, tolterodine[30]

When discontinued, anticholinergic medications should be stopped slowly and tapered as an abrupt discontinuation can cause withdrawal symptoms such as agitation, diarrhea, vomiting, lacrimation, tachycardia, insomnia, and movement disorders, leading to more discomfort for the patient.[30]

Analgesics

There are multiple reasons patients at nursing homes present for short- or long-term stay receive pain medications. Acetaminophen has evidence for safe alleviation of pain and augmenting pain relief in older adults. NSAIDs may also be effective at treating chronic pain from a medical condition such as arthritis, but preferably topical over systemic. Long-term use of NSAIDs in the elderly is concerning for gastric ulcers and worsening of heart failure, hypertension, and kidney disease. Opioids should be used in situations after non-opioid medications have been used. Opioids may be needed to achieve functional independence that cannot be done by other interventions. When deprescribing opioids used for acute pain relief, if used as needed and minimally, these medications can be stopped. For those who have been on a scheduled regular regimen, opioids can be decreased each week by 10% to 50%. If the patient shows withdrawal symptoms or worsening pain, tapering should be paused or the dose should be returned to the previous dose for appropriate pain control.[18]

Constipation Medications

Constipation and other gastrointestinal symptoms are leading contributors to polypharmacy in nursing home patients. With a combination of decreased fluid intake, reduced ADL, lack of movement and exercise, side effects from medications, and neurologic and metabolic disorders, nursing home patients are at high risk of constipation. A cross-sectional study in Norway nursing homes discovered that rather than polypharmacy, constipation was associated with specific groups of drugs such as BZRAs, antidepressants, opioids, propionic acid derivatives or NSAIDs, and anticholinergic medications.[31] In an Italian retrospective cross-sectional multicenter study, antidepressants, anti-Parkinson dopaminergic medications, and benzodiazepines were commonly used with laxatives .

Reviewing the side effects of medications is most important when handling polypharmacy and constipation. Laxatives are a frequent subject of the prescribing cascade.[32] When patients require medications with a known or anticipated side effect of constipation, it is appropriate to provide medications to help with constipation. However, once the medication with constipation as a side effect is stopped, medications prescribed for constipation should also be reviewed and stopped when appropriate.

Proton-Pump Inhibitors

PPIs also frequently contribute to polypharmacy in the nursing home. In an Italy-based multicenter observational study, 50% of nursing home patients were taking PPIs for evidence-based indications. Corticosteroids, anticoagulants, and mean number of medications were important predictors of inappropriate use. Residents who received 13 medications or more were about 10 times higher risk of receiving a PPI than those on 0 to 4 medications.

One small pilot study created and implemented a nursing home stepwise taper protocol for PPIs. Every 3 weeks the dose of PPI was decreased by half and then the PPI was given every other day. On stopping the PPI, a histamine receptor antagonist was given and tapered off with the same discontinuation protocol. In this study, 90% of patients were able to stop PPIs in a 12-week period and none of these patients needed an antacid, prokinetic, or antisecretory medication at the 4-week mark.[33] In a multicenter, longitudinal, single-arm study of nursing homes in the Netherlands, a deprescribing algorithm was used to successfully stop a PPI in 27 of 31 residents. Only two residents experienced a withdrawal effect, dyspepsia, which resolved after restarting the PPI at a lower dose. Unsuccessful deprescribing was due to a valid indication for the PPI, such as GI bleeding or patient preference to continue the medication.[12]

Hypertension Medications

In an observational study of Medicare-enrolled US nursing home residents, more intensive antihypertensive treatment was associated with a small increase in hospitalizations and decrease in ADL decline after adjusting for physical function, prognosis, comorbid conditions, and age. However, there was no difference in mortality. Overall, there were no significant benefits from intensive antihypertensive treatment.[34]

The 8th Joint National Committee on Hypertension recommends treating hypertension in adults age 60 years or older with a target of < 150/90. Although tight blood pressure control may decrease cardiovascular risk, many studies that support intense blood pressure control have been done in ambulatory, healthier individuals. More studies are needed in nursing home patients, focusing on whether strict blood pressure control has impact on cardiovascular, hospitalizations, mortality risks and whether less antihypertensive medications decrease adverse events.[34,35]

Diabetic Medications

Diabetes in older adults has been linked to higher mortality, increased institutionalization, and reduction in functional status. Higher A1C goals, less than 8.5%, are reasonable for those with more comorbid conditions and shorter estimated life expectancy. Except for metformin, which provides long-term reductions in myocardial infarction and mortality, using other medications to achieve A1C levels less than 7% may be associated with more harm and higher mortality rate. There is a small amount of cardiovascular and microvascular benefit in those with multiple medical conditions and strict A1C goals. The U-shaped relationship between mortality and A1C has been reported, with higher mortality rates seen in those with A1C less than 6% and greater than 8.5% to 11%. With deprescribing, there is a low risk for rebound hyperglycemia in those that already have a low or within goal A1C.[36,37] The American Diabetes Association suggests to avoid relying on A1C in the nursing home and instead monitor using blood glucose, with the target of 100-200 mg/dL. In nursing homes, diabetic medications should be prescribed based on hypoglycemia risk with the focus on simplifying the medication regimen and avoiding sole use of sliding scale insulin.[38,39]

Statins

In frail older adults, statins can be safe and should not be discontinued solely due to increasing age. Statins and their use or discontinuation should be individualized, taking into consideration life expectancy, side effects, and possible drug–drug interactions. Starting statins in individuals 80 years and older is usually considered for secondary prevention in patients with atherosclerotic cardiovascular disease (ASCVD) and a life expectancy of more than 5 years. If a patient does not have clear evidence of ASCVD, the provider should consider and discuss with the patient whether to discontinue the statin.[40] Unfortunately, U.S. guidelines for prescribing statins in older adults are inconsistent. Studies have shown that statins are not helpful and contribute to the therapeutic burden of older adults near end of life. Deprescribing statins has not been shown to increase mortality for older adults with ASCVD. Thus, the American Medical Directors Association recommends against routine prescribing of lipid-lowering agents for older patients with limited life expectancies.[41]

Anticoagulation

Older adults in nursing homes are recommended to have anticoagulation when they are at increased risk of stroke due to the debilitating sequelae of a major stroke. In general, for nursing home patients in the setting of polypharmacy, direct oral anticoagulants (DOACs) can be preferred as warfarin has more drug–drug interactions and blood work monitoring. For those that have increased benefit with frequent monitoring, appropriately managed warfarin may be preferred. Overall, there is not a lot of information on the safety and efficacy of warfarin and DOACs in the very old patients. However, owing to increasing availability of DOACs and less required monitoring and known drug–drug interactions, more nursing home residents are being prescribed DOACs. More evidence is needed for use of DOACs specific to nursing home residents and whether anticoagulants have benefits that outweigh risks, especially in residents with significant cognitive and physical impairment.[42]

Acetylcholinesterase Inhibitors

AChEIs are usually prescribed for stabilization or decreased rate of decline in cognitive, behavioral, or functional symptoms in patients with dementia.[17,43] The American Geriatrics Society states that AChEI may lead to improvement in cognitive testing results, however, there is no clear evidence that there is delayed institutionalization, improved quality of life, or decreased burden on caregivers. If the desired effect is not seen in approximately 3 months, the AChEI should be discontinued.[36] Side effects include negative gastrointestinal and urinary symptoms, weight loss, and syncope, all of which may have detrimental effects on the quality of life in the frail older adults at the nursing home. One of the main barriers to deprescribing AChEI is the potential worsening of behavioral symptoms. Yet, in severe dementia, studies show that worsening behavioral symptoms of these medications are not clinically significant. In a national sample of U.S. nursing home residents with severe dementia, deprescribing AChEIs was not associated with all-cause negative events and rather associated with reduced likelihood of hospitalization due to falls or fractures.[43]

In a retrospective analysis of Medicare data, AChEI discontinuation was more likely in patients with a limited prognosis, especially those with severe dementia and life expectancy of 6 months or less. Discontinuation occurred more frequently in admission assessments compared with quarterly or annual assessments. Residents in nursing homes in rural areas were associated with decreased likelihood of discontinuation of AChEI compared with urban areas. Geriatricians were also more likely to deprescribe AChEI compared with general practitioners, possibly due to increased knowledge of medications and ADRs in older adults.[44]

BARRIERS TO DEPRESCRIBING

Major themes of barriers to deprescribing are operations and routines, resources and qualifications, patient-related outcomes, policies, and collaboration and communication.[28] Reasons also arise from the clinician, patient, and those involved in the patient's decision-making. There may be pressure to prescribe evoked by recommendations contained within disease-specific clinical guidelines. Many of these recommendations are less applicable and relevant in the older, multimorbid patient population. A large number of clinical trials providing evidence for such guidelines have criteria that exclude frail older adults from their studies.[45] Current interventions have led to identification and resolution of medication-related problems and improvements in medication appropriateness. More research evaluating clinical outcomes of deprescribing, particularly specific to nursing home patients is needed to support guidelines to address polypharmacy in the nursing home.

Despite the barriers, the key to addressing polypharmacy in nursing homes is ongoing discussions with the patient or the patient's decision maker regarding the patient's goals. By ensuring that the patient's goals are clear, whether it may be to optimize medical treatment for multiple chronic conditions or minimize medications for the purpose of preference and comfort, the provider can use this knowledge and the premise of providing benefit over harm as a guide for the treatment plan. Each patient represents an individualized case, and expert clinical knowledge is important. Ultimately, there should be a shared decision-making process and discussion with treatment team members and relevant subspecialists regarding patient's goals for successful prescribing and deprescribing.[45]

SUMMARY

Polypharmacy is a concern for the growing number of older adults in the nursing home, especially as these older adults are frail and have more comorbidities. Medications that should be reviewed when addressing polypharmacy include frequently prescribed medications in the nursing home such as gastrointestinal, psychiatric, and pain medications, medications prescribed in common comorbidities, and medications with particularly adverse side effects such as anticholinergic medications. Important periods in which medication review is essential include admission to the nursing home and with any major medical changes. Deprescribing medications is a complex task that is best achieved in collaboration with all members of the care team and the patient. With successful deprescribing, better overall health outcomes can be achieved for nursing home residents.

CLINICS CARE POINTS

- In long-term care, nursing homes have the highest prevalence of older adults with Alzheimer's disease. Frail nursing home residents, especially those with dementia, are more likely to be started on potentially inappropriate medications and less likely to have them discontinued.

- Several important medication classes are inappropriately prescribed in the nursing home. Medications should be reviewed for appropriateness based on criteria discussed in this article.

- The Screening Tool of Older Person's Prescriptions and Screening Tools to Alert Doctors to Right Treatment (STOPP and START) criteria, when used in nursing homes, led to patients receiving fewer medications, less frequent falls, and lower medication costs.

- Deprescribing in the nursing home population led to a significantly reduced number of residents with potentially inappropriate medications; specifically medication review-directed deprescribing interventions led to reduction of all-cause mortality and reduction in the number of falls.

DISCLOSURE

The authors have nothing to disclose.

REFERENCES

1. Harper GM, Lyons WL, Potter JF, editors. Geriatrics review syllabus: a core curriculum in geriatric medicine. 10th edition. New York, N.Y.: American Geriatrics Society; 2019. p. 218–30.
2. Payne RA. The epidemiology of polypharmacy. Clin Med (Lond) 2016;16(5): 465–9.
3. Tamura BK, Bell CL, Inaba M, et al. Outcomes of polypharmacy in nursing home residents. Clin Geriatr Med 2012;28(2):217–36.
4. Centers for Medicare & Medicaid Services. Nursing home data compendium 2015 edition. HHS Guidance Repository; 2020.
5. Burt J, Elmore N, Campbell SM, et al. Developing a measure of polypharmacy appropriateness in primary care: systematic review and expert consensus study. BMC Med 2018;16(1):91. Published 2018 Jun 13.

6. Harris-Kojetin L, Sengupta M, Lendon JP, et al. Long-term care providers and services users in the United States, 2015–2016. National Center for Health Statistics. Vital Health Stat 2019;3(43).

7. Dwyer LL, Han B, Woodwell DA, et al. Polypharmacy in nursing home residents in the United States: results of the 2004 national nursing home survey. Am J Geriatr Pharmacother 2010;8(1):63–72.

8. Davies EA, O'Mahony MS. Adverse drug reactions in special populations - the elderly. Br J Clin Pharmacol 2015;80(4):796–807.

9. Wastesson JW, Morin L, Tan ECK, et al. An update on the clinical consequences of polypharmacy in older adults: a narrative review. Expert Opin Drug Saf 2018; 17(12):1185–96.

10. Maclagan LC, Maxwell CJ, Gandhi S, et al. Frailty and potentially inappropriate medication use at nursing home transition. J Am Geriatr Soc 2017;65(10): 2205–12.

11. Chhabra PT, Rattinger GB, Dutcher SK, et al. Medication reconciliation during the transition to and from long-term care settings: a systematic review. Res Social Adm Pharm 2012;8(1):60–75.

12. Visser AGR, Schols JMGA, Prevoo MALM, et al. Deprescribing statins and proton pump inhibitors in nursing home residents; a pragmatic exploratory study. Gerontol Geriatr Med 2021;7. 23337214211050807.

13. By the 2019 American Geriatrics Society Beers Criteria® Update Expert Panel. American geriatrics society 2019 updated ags beers criteria® for potentially inappropriate medication use in older adults. J Am Geriatr Soc 2019;67(4): 674–94.

14. Khodyakov D, Ochoa A, Olivieri-Mui BL, et al. Screening tool of older person's prescriptions/screening tools to alert doctors to right treatment medication criteria modified for U.S. nursing home setting. J Am Geriatr Soc 2017;65(3):586–91.

15. O'Mahony D. STOPP/START criteria for potentially inappropriate medications/potential prescribing omissions in older people: origin and progress. Expert Rev Clin Pharmacol 2020;13(1):15–22.

16. Thompson W, Farrell B. Deprescribing: what is it and what does the evidence tell us? Can J Hosp Pharm 2013;66(3):201–2.

17. Deprescribing guidelines and algorithms. Available at: https://deprescribing.org/. https://deprescribing.org/resources/deprescribing-guidelines-algorithms/. Accessed January 2022.

18. Hoel RW, Giddings Connolly RM, Takahashi PY. Polypharmacy management in older patients. Mayo Clin Proc 2021;96(1):242–56.

19. Kua CH, Mak VSL, Huey Lee SW. Health Outcomes of deprescribing interventions among older residents in nursing homes: a systematic review and meta-analysis. J Am Med Dir Assoc 2019;20(3):362–72.e11.

20. Farrell B, Mangin D. Deprescribing is an essential part of good prescribing. Am Fam Physician 2019;99(1):7–9.

21. Maust DT, Langa KM, Blow FC, et al. Psychotropic use and associated neuropsychiatric symptoms among patients with dementia in the USA. Int J Geriatr Psychiatry 2017;32(2):164–74.

22. Hanlon JT, Handler SM, Castle NG. Antidepressant prescribing in US nursing homes between 1996 and 2006 and its relationship to staffing patterns and use of other psychotropic medications. J Am Med Dir Assoc 2010;11(5):320–4.

23. Thakur M, Blazer DG. Depression in long-term care. J Am Med Dir Assoc 2008; 9(2):82–7.

24. Bourgeois J, Elseviers MM, Van Bortel L, et al. The use of antidepressants in Belgian nursing homes: focus on indications and dosages in the PHEBE study. Drugs Aging 2012;29(9):759–69.

25. Guina J, Merrill B. Benzodiazepines I: upping the care on downers: the evidence of risks, benefits and alternatives. J Clin Med 2018;7(2):17. Published 2018 Jan 30.

26. Rijksen DOC, Zuidema SU, de Haas EC. Use of benzodiazepines and Z-drugs in nursing home residents with dementia: prevalence and appropriateness. J Alzheimers Dis Rep 2021;5(1):871–9. Published 2021 Dec 9.

27. Chiu Y, Bero L, Hessol NA, et al. A literature review of clinical outcomes associated with antipsychotic medication use in North American nursing home residents. Health Policy 2015;119(6):802–13.

28. Moth AE, Hølmkjær P, Holm A, et al. What makes deprescription of psychotropic drugs in nursing home residents with dementia so challenging? a qualitative systematic review of barriers and facilitators. Drugs Aging 2021;38(8):671–85.

29. Chatterjee S, Bali V, Carnahan RM, et al. Anticholinergic burden and risk of cognitive impairment in elderly nursing home residents with depression. Res Social Adm Pharm 2020;16(3):329–35.

30. López-Álvarez J, Sevilla-Llewellyn-Jones J, Agüera-Ortiz L. Anticholinergic drugs in geriatric psychopharmacology. Front Neurosci 2019;13:1309.

31. Fosnes GS, Lydersen S, Farup PG. Drugs and constipation in elderly in nursing homes: what is the relation? Gastroenterol Res Pract 2012;2012:290231.

32. Elli C, Novella A, Nobili A, et al. Laxative agents in nursing homes: an example of prescribing cascade. J Am Med Dir Assoc 2021;22(12):2559–64.

33. Farrell B, Pottie K, Thompson W, et al. Deprescribing proton pump inhibitors: evidence-based clinical practice guideline. Can Fam Physician 2017;63(5):354–64.

34. Boockvar KS, Song W, Lee S, et al. Hypertension treatment in us long-term nursing home residents with and without dementia. J Am Geriatr Soc 2019;67(10):2058–64.

35. Vu M, Schleiden LJ, Harlan ML, et al. Hypertension management in nursing homes: review of evidence and considerations for care. Curr Hypertens Rep 2020;22(1):8. Published 2020 Jan 14.

36. American Geriatrics Society. Ten things clinicians and patients should question. choosing wisely. Available at: https://www.choosingwisely.org/societies/american-geriatrics-society/. Accessed January 2022.

37. Aspinall SL, Hanlon JT, Niznik JD, et al. Deprescribing in older nursing home patients: focus on innovative composite measures for dosage deintensification. Innov Aging 2017;1(2):igx031. Published 2017 Dec 20.

38. Munshi MN, Florez H, Huang ES, et al. Management of diabetes in long-term care and skilled nursing facilities: a position statement of the american diabetes association. Diabetes Care 2016;39(2):308–18.

39. American Diabetes Association Professional Practice Committee. 13. Older Adults: Standards of Medical Care in Diabetes—2022. Diabetes Care 2022;45(1):195–207. https://doi.org/10.2337/dc22-S013.

40. Benetos A, Rossignol P, Cherubini A, et al. Polypharmacy in the aging patient: management of hypertension in octogenarians [published correction appears in JAMA. JAMA 2015;314(6):628.

41. Mack DS, Tjia J, Hume AL, et al. Prevalent statin use in long-stay nursing home residents with life-limiting illness. J Am Geriatr Soc 2020;68(4):708–16.

42. Alcusky M, Lapane KL. Treatment of atrial fibrillation in nursing homes: a place for direct acting oral anticoagulants? J Nurs Home Res Sci 2018;4:15–9.

43. Niznik JD, Zhao X, He M, et al. Risk for health events after deprescribing acetylcholinesterase inhibitors in nursing home residents with severe dementia. J Am Geriatr Soc 2020;68(4):699–707.

44. Niznik JD, Zhao X, He M, et al. Factors associated with deprescribing acetylcholinesterase inhibitors in older nursing home residents with severe dementia. J Am Geriatr Soc 2019;67(9):1871–9.

45. Lun P, Tang JY, Lee JQ, et al. Barriers to appropriate prescribing in older adults with multimorbidity: a modified Delphi study. Aging Med (Milton) 2021;4(3): 180–92.

Polypharmacy in the Hospitalized Older Adult

Considerations for Safe and Effective Treatment

Analiese DiConti-Gibbs, MD[a],*, Kimberly Y Chen, DO[b,c],
Charles Edward Coffey Jr, MD, MS[d,e]

KEYWORDS

- Polypharmacy • Hospital • Deprescribing • Geriatrics • Comorbidity

KEY POINTS

- Polypharmacy is a common and risky occurrence for older adults.
- Hospitalization provides a key opportunity to keep older adults safe by reducing polypharmacy and mitigating risks in key clinical scenarios
- Rigorous attention to detail during transitions of care is key to reducing the risk older adults experience from polypharmacy

Abbreviations	
ACE	Angiotensin Converting Enzyme
ARB	Angiotensin Receptor Blocker
UTI	Urinary Tract Infection

INTRODUCTION

Care for the older adult is growing ever more complex. As a result, 91% of older adults regularly take one or more medications per day and 43% take five of more.[1] Though these medications may help primary conditions, they create polypharmacy and place the patient at risk for adverse drug events (ADEs). This article reviews polypharmacy in the hospitalized older adult from admission to discharge and offers key tools and resources for clinicians to use to keep patients safe from the ill effects of polypharmacy.

[a] Division of Geriatrics, Hospital, Palliative, and General Internal Medicine, Keck School of Medicine of USC, 2020 Zonal Ave, IRD 306, Los Angeles, CA 90033; [b] Primary Care, Welbe Pacific/PACE, 50 Alessandro Place, A20, Pasadena, CA 91105, USA; [c] LAC+USC/Keck School of Medicine Geriatric Fellowship, 2020 Zonal Ave, IRD 306, Los Angeles, CA, 90033; [d] LAC+USC Medical Center, Suite C2K100, Room 115, 2051 Marengo Street, Los Angeles, CA 90033, USA; [e] Keck School of Medicine of USC, 1975 Zonal Ave, Los Angeles, CA 90033
* Corresponding author. LAC+USC Medical Center/Keck School of Medicine of USC, GHPGIM, 2020 Zonal Ave, IRD 306, Los Angeles, CA 90033
E-mail address: Analiese.diconti-gibbs@med.usc.edu

Clin Geriatr Med 38 (2022) 667–684
https://doi.org/10.1016/j.cger.2022.07.011
0749-0690/22/© 2022 Elsevier Inc. All rights reserved.
geriatric.theclinics.com

EMERGENCY ROOM AND ADMISSION

Older adults are visiting emergency departments (EDs) and being hospitalized at a higher rate than ever before. Adults over 65 year old account for 19.6 million ED visits from 2009 to 2010 in the United States, which was 15% of all ED visits.[2] The percentage of ED visits that resulted in hospital admission increased with age: 32.4% for ages 65% to 74%, 37.2% for ages 75% to 84%, and 43.4% for those 85 and over.[2] Patients admitted to the hospital provide an opportunity to review the dosing, indications, and necessity for prescribed medications, with a keen eye to reduce polypharmacy.

Admissions Due to Adverse Drug Events

As polypharmacy grows in prevalence, so do hospitalizations due to ADEs. In 2013 to 2014, population rates for ED visits for ADEs were 9.7 per 1000 individuals among adults 65 years or older, with a hospitalization rate of 44% for these visits,[3] compared with just 10% of admissions for older adults during 1988 to 2015.[4] When adjusted for population, the hospitalization rate for older adults due to ADEs was seven times the rate of those younger than 65 years.[3]

Oscanoa and colleagues[4] reviewed common medications causing hospital admission for ADEs from 1988 to 2015. In this meta-analysis, nonsteroidal anti-inflammatory drugs (NSAIDs) were responsible for 10% of admissions. Common medications and their rate and reason for admissions can be seen in **Table 1**.

Table 1
Frequent medications associated with emergency room visits due to ADEs based on meta-analysis[4]

Drug Class	Proportion of Emergency Room Visits	Clinical Presentations
NSAIDs	2.3%–33%	Upper gastrointestinal bleed, renal failure, coronary events, and hypertension
Beta blockers	1%–14.5%	Syncope, bradycardia, heart block, hypotension, and falls
Antibiotics	1.1%–22.2%	Diarrhea, vomiting, renal failure, *Clostridium difficile* infection, hypersensitivity, urticaria, seizures, and Stevens–Johnson syndrome
Warfarin	3.3%–55.6%	INR increase, anemia, gastrointestinal bleed, bleeding, and dyspnea
Digoxin	1.6%–18.8%	Bradycardia, heart block, cardiac arrhythmias, syncope, nausea, vomiting, delirium, heart failure, and poor appetite
ACE inhibitors	5.5%–23.4%	Hyponatremia, hyperkalemia, hypotension, fall, acute kidney injury, cough, syncope, and neutropenia
Antitumorals	1.5%–9.1%	Anemia, fall, pancytopenia, fever, diarrhea, vomiting, and skin rash
Calcium-entry blockers	1%–8.5%	Syncope, bradycardia, heart failure, fall, hypotension, cardiac arrhythmias, edema, and hypotonia
Opioids	1.5%–18.8%	Fall, mental status changes, GI disturbances, confusion, somnolence, vertigo/fracture, hallucinations, constipation
Antidiabetics	4.5%–22.2%	Hypoglycemia, acidosis, altered mental status, and fatigue

Many ADEs are dose-related,[4,5] so using the mantra "start low and go slow" may prevent many hospitalizations due to ADEs. Polypharmacy also increases the risk of drug-drug interactions (DDIs), which often present as nonspecific symptoms (eg, fatigue, nausea, depression, confusion, or appetite loss).[5] Computer-based algorithms to reduce polypharmacy on admission have been tried but have had poor uptake by providers and have not shown efficacy.[6] For patients admitted with an ADE, clinicians should carefully review whether the offending medication should be continued, dose-reduced, or stopped altogether.

Medication Reconciliation

Medication reconciliation by the admitting clinician ensures safe medication use during hospitalization. A thorough medication review will cross-check medications against other patient data, including morbidities, patient's preferences, or geriatric syndromes, to produce a personalized medication strategy.[7] In addition, a hospital admission may provide new information about a patient's health, including new diagnoses, that will require a change in medication regimen. Inclusion of hospital pharmacists in the reconciliation process improves the identification of potential drug-related problems.[8] Multiple tools exist to help the medical team determine potentially inappropriate medications (PIMs), which will be discussed later in this article.

Over the Counter Supplements and Herbal Medications

Though there's little evidence of benefit for many of the supplements patients take, dietary supplements, including multi-vitamins, are widely used by older adults. Often clinicians find multiple supplements or herbal medications during medication reconciliation. These supplements may have been recommended by a medical provider or may have been selected by the patient or family for a perceived health benefit. The US Preventative Service Task Force concluded that current evidence is insufficient to assess the balance of benefits and harms of the use of multivitamin supplements for the prevention of cardiovascular disease or cancer,[9] which patients often report as the reason for supplement use. Self-prescribed supplement use has many risks like misdiagnosis, wrong drug dosage, prolonged duration of use, drug interactions, and polypharmacy.[10] Furthermore, adverse events related to supplements cause over 23,000 ED visits per year in the United States.[11] Clinicians should ask patients about supplement use, as supplements may be targets for deprescribing.[12]

As many supplements and herbal medications have multiple ingredients and may not be tested for accuracy of dosage information, clinicians must work with patients to choose products that have been tested by independent agencies to maximize safety. Yet making decisions on deprescribing and risk/benefit analyses is quite difficult. Clinicians can use resources like Stockley's Herbal Medicines Interactions and Herbalbase, an independent Finnish database of evidence-based information on herbal medications that is continually updated, to research supplements and guide their discussion with patients.[13]

HOSPITALIZATION

Annually there are 13.2 million hospitalizations in adults 65 years and older[14] and up to 45% of these patients are discharged on five or more medications.[15] Over two-thirds of Medicare beneficiaries have two or more chronic conditions and 40% have four or more.[16] Many older adults are admitted to the general medical service for one of many chronic conditions, including hypertension, heart disease, diabetes, kidney disease, and chronic obstructive pulmonary disease (COPD).[16] Unfortunately, many chronic medical conditions are best treated with multiple medications, thereby increasing the risk of ADEs and polypharmacy. Thus, the hospitalization of an older adult is an opportunity for providers to review their conditions, medications, and their indications, and engage in shared decision-making with patients about their mediations. In this section, we review the concerns, risks, and opportunities to improve polypharmacy in various medical conditions so that clinicians will be best prepared to discuss risks, benefits, and alternatives with hospitalized older adults.

Anticoagulation and Bleeding

The most common reasons for anticoagulation prescription in hospitalized patients are prevention or treatment of venous thromboembolism, atrial fibrillation, and stroke or cardiac event. Age is a risk factor not only for stroke and thromboembolism but also for bleeding, as pathophysiological changes occur that alter drug kinetics and toxicity of oral anticoagulants at standard doses.[17] In addition, the higher clinical complexity of older patients (a.k.a. multimorbidity) complicates the decision whether to anticoagulated, as multimorbidity both increases risk of stroke without anticogulation[18] and is a risk factor for bleeding and ADEs. Warfarin was the most common cause of hospitalizations due to an ADE at more than 30,000 hospitalizations annually.[19] Target-specific oral anticoagulants were associated with a lower risk for stroke and intracranial hemorrhage but have a higher risk of gastrointestinal bleed when compared with warfarin.[20] Overall, the absolute benefits of anticoagulants increase with older age and additional stroke risk factors, so providers should work with patients to determine whether the benefits of anticoagulants are worth increased bleeding risk, potential DDIs, and increased complexity of clinical management.[18] Patients should be counseled to wear an alert bracelet, keep an updated and accurate medication list, and ensure familiarity with medications in case of emergencies.[18]

Congestive Heart Failure

Patients with congestive heart failure (CHF) on Guideline-Directed Medical Therapy (GDMT) frequently experience polypharmacy. GDMT includes at least three different medications, and up to ten different classes of medications which may be variably prescribed depending on symptomatology and severity.[21] In addition, over 60% of Medicare beneficiaries with the diagnosis of CHF have five or more other chronic conditions that contribute to this polypharmacy,[16] and 95% of patients with CHF are discharged with five or more medications.[22] The number of patients hospitalized for CHF taking ten or more medications increased between the periods of 2003 to 2006 and 2011 to 2014: 25% versus 55% of patients, respectively; interestingly, the increase in medications was greatest in non-cardiovascular medications.[22]

The most common medications started during hospitalization for CHF are loop diuretics (27%), beta-blockers (21%), aspirin (19%), electrolyte supplements (17%), ACE inhibitors (17%), Quinolones (12%), Anticoagulants (12%), Proton pump inhibitors (11%), and statins (11%).[22] Although many of these medications are part of GDMT with clear benefits to morbidity or mortality, the benefit of starting medications other than GDMT is debatable. Clinicians should carefully assess the risks, benefits, and alternatives to non-GDMT medications to minimize ADEs from polypharmacy. Common side effects of GDMT include:

- Beta-blockers: weakness/fatigue (19%), syncope (17%), hypotension (13%), worsening heart failure (5%), and bradycardia (4%).[23]
- ACE inhibitors and ARBs: symptomatic first-dose hypotension (3%)[24] but no statistically significant long-term effect in GFR.[25]

- Spironolactone: hyperkalemia greater than 5.5 mmol/L, acute kidney injury, and discontinuation of therapy depending on the study population.[23]
- Digoxin: toxicity common in doses above 0.25 mg, in patients with serum creatinine above 120 mcg/L, or with coadministration of amiodarone, propafenone, quinidine, or verapamil.[23]

Given most patients with CHF take at least five medications, clinicians can consider these patients having high-risk polypharmacy if they are prescribed 10 or more medications.[22] GDMT can add years to the life of a patient with CHF and prevent over 10,000 deaths per year in the United States,[26] but clinicians must assess the risk of polypharmacy and ADEs, as clinical trial data on medication efficacy and safety routinely exclude patients most vulnerable to these side effects.[27] Clinicians may take a balanced approach in this assessment to include the patient's functional status and frailty as well as their life goals, and social environment. Once GMDT is started, clinicians must monitor patients closely for both effectiveness (eg, weight, urine output, blood pressure) and side effect profile (hypotension, bradycardia, dizziness). Patients should also be counseled on expected versus concerning side effects that require urgent evaluation and strategies to manage expected side effects.

Chronic Obstructive Pulmonary Disease

Most clinicians follow the GOLD strategy for treating COPD in the inpatient setting.[28] When stepping up COPD care, home medication doses are often increased rather than new medications added. As such, COPD treatment infrequently causes polypharmacy. The most common additional medications prescribed for COPD exacerbations are antibiotics and steroids, usually for a week-long course.[29] An important COPD treatment adjunct that adds to polypharmacy are therapies to combat nicotine dependence, including varenicline, bupropion, nortriptyline, and nicotine replacements (eg, gum, inhalers, nasal spray, and patches). Polypharmacy may also increase for patients who get their COPD medications from inpatient pharmacies at discharge, as formulary issues force many hospital pharmacies to break combination inhalers to their component inhalers, thereby increasing medications and potential patient confusion upon discharge. Unfortunately, adherence to COPD medication regimen is poor for most patients, and is worse with polypharmacy, leading to frequent rehospitalizations for exacerbations.[30]

Pulmonary rehabilitation is a good non-pharmacologic option available to optimize breathing comfort and oxygen exchange and symptomatically relieve dyspnea and fatigue, reaffirms autonomy over disease progression, and improves emotional processing of hospitalization.[31] Immunization for influenza and pneumococcal disease can also reduce hospitalizations and thus new medication prescriptions in the COPD population.[32]

Infections

Infections commonly plague hospitalized older adults due to immunocompromise, decreased physiologic reserve, and skin barrier breakdown that occurs with aging. Treatment of infections in older adults often requires at least one medication, thereby contributing to polypharmacy and the risk of ADEs.

For example, Noor and colleagues[33] found that 73% of patients admitted with pneumonia, had a potential DDI, over half of which were classified as "major". The most frequent DDIs noted were decreased therapeutic response, electrolyte abnormalities, hypoglycemia, bleeding, hepatotoxicity, and hypertension. And unsurprisingly, the risk of potential DDIs increased with number of drugs prescribed.[33] Antibiotics associated with hypoglycemia include fluoroquinolones, clarithromycin, linezolid, tige-cycline, cefditoren, doxycycline, trimethoprim-sulfamethoxazole.[34] To complicate matters, clinicians often stop oral antihyperglycemics in favor of subcutaneous insulin for hospitalized patients. On discharge, oral antibiotics and oral antihyperglycemics combined may cause more frequent and severe episodes of hypoglycemia.

Beyond ADEs and DDIs, polypharmacy is an independent predictor of treatment outcomes in UTIs.[35] Specifically, patients taking medications like loop diuretics, thia-zides, and ACE inhibitors reported increased urinary symptoms that resolved with medications cessation. Patients taking loop diuretics have increased urinary fre-quency and relaxation of the bladder that reduced the risk of UTI, whereas medica-tions reducing urinary incontinence can increase the frequency of UTIs. Patients taking ACE inhibitors have increased stress incontinence with cough and reported more frequent UTI symptoms.[35] Diagnosis of UTIs in older adults can be difficult as diagnosis depends on symptomatology, and polypharmacy confounds many urinary symptoms.

In patients admitted with coronavirus disease-2019 (COVID-19) positivity, polyphar-macy was associated with increased death among male patients, increased rate of acute kidney injury, and ADEs.[36] Antipsychotic drugs specifically were associated with almost a three times risk of severe COVID-19 morbidity and an increased risk of death above COVID-19-infected men (71%) and women (96%).[36]

Chronic Kidney Disease and Kidney Failure

Polypharmacy is common in patients with chronic kidney disease (CKD) and causes significant morbidity and mortality. A study in Japan estimated the prevalence of poly-pharmacy in this population at 38%, and found that patients taking more than ten medications had the highest risk of kidney failure, cardiovascular events, and all-cause mortality.[37] Patients on five to nine medications had an increased risk of kidney failure compared with those on less than five medications.[37] A large US study showed increased mortality in patients with polypharmacy and CKD (hazard ratio [HR] 1.22–2.35).[38] ADEs are common and often serious in patients with CKD. Renin-angiotensin system inhibitors, antithrombotic agents, and diuretics are the most com-mon medications to cause ADEs in this population, but anticoagulants cause 34% of serious complications.[39] In patients with CKD taking more than five medications, those with eGFR less than 30 had a significantly higher risk for ADEs.[39] Pharmacists are key to improving medication safety for patients with CKD and can help clinicians deprescribe and dose-adjust medications based on GFR. Sadly, clinicians follow less than 50% of the pharmacists' recommendations.[40]

Diabetes

Polypharmacy is common in the management of hyperglycemia and the numerous microvascular (diabetic nephropathy, neuropathy, retinopathy), macrovascular complications (coronary artery disease, peripheral arterial disease, stroke), geriatric syndromes associated with diabetes (cognitive impairment, falls, urinary inconti-nence).[41] Yet, antidiabetic medications also increase the risk of hypoglycemia, falls, fractures, impaired cognitive performance, heart failure, urinary incontinence, and UTIs in the diabetic older adult.[41] The balance of managing diabetes and hypergly-cemia while minimizing adverse events is challenging, especially in the hospital setting.

In the hospitalized patient, the target blood sugar range is 140 to 180 mg/dL.[42] To achieve this narrow target, clinicians often use subcutaneous insulin instead of oral antihyperglycemic medications. Insulin-based medication regimens often result in clinicians missing DDIs between new medications and the oral antihyperglycemic medications the patient takes at home. In addition, acute illness can change a patient's insulin needs as hyper- or hypoglycemia can be induced in the acute setting and may persist in the early post-discharge period. Antihyperglycemic regimens prescribed post-discharge should be clearly written out and verbal instructions with a teach-back technique should be given to the patient to ensure understanding. Close primary care follow-up on discharge is also recommended for patients whose antihyperglycemic needs are expected to change.

Deprescribing in the Hospital Setting

Deprescribing medications in the hospital setting is challenging. First, patients may be resistant to changes made by an unfamiliar hospital-based clinician instead of their primary care provider with whom they have rapport. Second, each admission may bring new diagnoses and new medications. Hospital-based clinicians should engage in shared decision-making with the patient and their primary care provider whenever possible. Providers seeking to deprescribe should follow a systematic approach to deprescribing, including:

- Document a clear indication or diagnosis associated with each medication the patient is currently taking.
- Identify PIMs the patient may be taking.
- If the medication can be deprescribed, determine whether it requires tapering and/or monitoring.
- Identify the provider that can follow up tapering and/or deprescribing.
- Review patient and caregiver preferences for medication regimen after the presentation of recommendations of the care team.[43,44]

To date, randomized control trials of deprescribing interventions have shown a reduction of pill burden but no statistically significant difference in drug-related problems, mortality, hospital readmissions, falls and functional status.[45,46] Risks of deprescribing interventions in the hospital setting include potential prescribing omissions that increased from 52.9% to 77.7%[47] and can lead to adverse outcomes.[48] Given the hospital team will only be providing care for a short time, patient and caregiver buy-in is critical to patient safety. In addition, follow-up by post-acute care or primary care providers to review or monitor response to medication changes is essential.

Perioperative Care

Approximately 33% of patients over 65 will undergo at least one surgical procedure before death.[49] Frequently perioperative evaluation and postoperative care unmask new medical conditions. For example, Sampson and colleagues[50] found that of patients over 70 year old admitted for emergency hospitalization 42.4% had dementia, 50% of which were undiagnosed before admission. It is important for all clinicians caring for older adults perioperatively, including hospitalists, surgeons, and the perioperative team, be familiar with issues facing older adults in the perioperative period.

American College of Surgeons and the American Geriatric Society published a joint best practice guidelines (American College of Surgeons National Surgical Quality Improvement Program [ACS NSQIP]/American Geriatrics Society [AGS] guidelines) to help guide physicians caring for the geriatric perioperative patient, many of which center on polypharmacy.[51,52] Recommendations include:

- Perform a thorough medication history including over-the-counter medications and supplements to inform anesthesiology about possible interactions.
- Discontinue nonessential medications perioperatively.
- Minimize the addition of new medications.
- Continue medications with withdrawal potential including selective serotonin reuptake inhibitors, tricyclic antidepressants, benzodiazepines, antipsychotics, monoamine-oxidase inhibitors, beta-blockers, clonidine, statins, and corticosteroids.
- Discontinue herbal medications at least 7 days before surgical operations due to the uncertainty of contents.

Patients with polypharmacy are often at high risk for delirium. Clinicians should use additional caution with anticholinergics and certain sedating medications. Antihistamine H1 antagonists such as diphenhydramine have strong anticholinergic effects and can trigger delirium. There is no conclusive evidence for H2 antagonists, tricyclic antidepressants, anti-Parkinsonians medications, steroids, NSAIDs, and antimuscarinics causing delirium. Fortunately, there is no increased risk associated with neuroleptics (antipsychotics) and digoxin.[51,52]

Hip Fractures

Hip fractures are more prevalent in patients with polypharmacy. Park and colleagues[53] found the odds ratio for hip fracture increased by level of polypharmacy: 1.65 odds ratio (OR) for patients taking 5 to 10 medications and 2.11 OR for patients taking greater than 10 medications when compared with a 0 to 1 medication group. This association is likely related to the fall risk of polypharmacy but may also speak to the frailty of patients who are susceptible to hip fracture. If hospitalized for hip fracture, the number of medications upon discharge is predictive of readmission but not death within 6 months after surgery.[54]

In the first month after surgery, patients could add 4 to 6 medications to their regular pill burden. Medications added commonly following hip fracture repair include anticoagulation, pain control, and osteoporosis treatment. Patients treated with anti-osteoporosis agents, SSRIs, and eye drops have an increased overall risk of readmission, whereas the use of vitamin K antagonists, thiazides, and tramadol is associated with an increased risk of readmission due to fall injury.[54] Though many of these medications are clearly indicated at discharge, many may have a safer alternative. Clinicians should carefully consider each patient's frailty and weigh this against the indication for each new drug prescribed; additional factors to consider include the patient and family's health literacy, discharge location, functional status, and fall risk.

Pain Control

Pain control in older adults is a complicated balance of achieving adequate pain control while minimizing side effects, DDIs and ADEs. Many providers are reluctant to treat pain aggressively due to these risks, but the postoperative patient has an increased risk of delirium from uncontrolled pain. Ideally, patients should be discharged with an uncomplicated pain control regimen that minimizes pill burden and risks to the patient. Common pain control agents and their risks and benefits are discussed in **Table 2**.

Medication regimen can be tailored based on the patient's comorbidities and potential for DDIs with their other medications. Ideally, pain control regimens should be time-limited and tapered to prevent persistent polypharmacy beyond the postoperative period.

Table 2
Risks and benefits of medications commonly used for postoperative pain control

Drug	Possible ADEs, Risks	Benefits	Recommendation
Acetaminophen and paracetamol	Hepatotoxicity[55]	Lower postoperative mortality[54] Reduced postoperative delirium[56,57] Reduced opioid use[56,57]	Maximal dose standing around the clock as a backbone of a postoperative pain control regimen
NSAIDs	Renal failure hypertension gastrointestinal bleed (GIB)[55,58]	Reduced inflammation Topical NSAIDs have added benefit when mixed with capsaicin or lidocaine cream[59]	Can be used short course inpatient in patients without known GIB risks or renal impairment[58] Daily evaluation of medical necessity and attempts to discontinue
Topical lidocaine	Contact dermatitis[60]	Minimal systemic effect	Beneficial for surgical site pain
Gabapentin and pregabalin	Dizziness, somnolence, and peripheral edema[60] Increased risk of overdose with opioids[55]	30%–50% pain abatement Improved sleep Fewer DDI[60]	Beneficial for surgical site and neuropathic pain
Duloxetine and venlafaxine	GI upset[55] DDIs with other protein-bound drugs[60]	No dose adjustment for age needed[60]	Beneficial for bony pain and neuropathic pain
Tramadol	Variable SNRI activity Associated with delirium[61]	Nocioceptive pain and neuropathic pain control	Should be avoided
Opioids	IV morphine increase postoperative mortality[54] Reduced respiratory drive, and increased delirium[55]	Effective pain control for visceral, nocioceptive, and neuropathic pain	Minimized but not avoided at the expense of uncontrolled pain postoperatively Use the lowest effective dose

Polypharmacy in the Intensive Care Unit

Polypharmacy is common for intensive care unit (ICU) patients, and older adults make up an increasing number of patients admitted to the ICU.[62] Older adults admitted to the ICU take an average of 12 different medications at the time of admission.[63] In addition to normal physiologic changes of aging, the acute organ dysfunction in critical illness may affect drug absorption, clearance, and physiologic response, and creating an increased risk for ADEs.[64] Several drugs commonly used to treat critical illness are listed in the Beers inventory of low benefit and/or high-risk medications, and the number of these medications prescribed is linearly correlated with length of stay.[65,66]

Intensive Care Unit Delirium

Polypharmacy is both a risk factor for and a sequela of delirium. Given the many confounding factors associated with critical illness, attributing an episode of ICU delirium to a specific medication is frequently a misplaced attribution.[67] Medications from most drug classes frequently given in the ICU may trigger delirium.[68] Medications most often attributed ICU delirium include anticholinergics and benzodiazepines.[69–71] Both Lorazepam and Midazolam were independently associated with a transition to delirium[69,70] and there is a 4% chance of delirium within the next hospital day for every 5 mg of midazolam given.[70] Delirium occurrence was only seen in 6% of cases in adults in the ICU in the day following the use of anticholinergic medications,[71] so it may not be as large of a factor in ICU delirium as previously thought. Medications given to treat agitated delirium, such as benzodiazepines, may also affect the mental status or lengthen the duration of delirium, and medications like antipsychotics are given off label to treat delirium to more than 10% of ICU patients.[67] Frequently, these medications are continued after the patient moves out of the ICU, further exacerbating polypharmacy, DDIs and ADEs.

To reduce polypharmacy in the delirious ICU patient, clinicians should treat delirium first with non-pharmacologic measures, such as:

- Screen patients regularly for pain, sedation, and delirium to quickly identify delirium-causing conditions and thus reduce pharmacologic delirium treatment.[67,72]
- Include friends and family in daily ICU care (eg, bathing, patient mobility exercises, and reorientation efforts).[67]
- Partner with a critical care pharmacist to conduct daily medication safety reviews and identify targets for deprescribing.[67]
- Conduct a preemptive evaluation of environmental and medication-related risk factors associated with delirium before pharmacologic interventions.[73]

Often pharmacologic treatment of delirium is needed given the time and effort associated with nonpharmacologic interventions. If medications are needed, clinicians should conduct daily medication reviews and attempt to discontinue or taper high-risk medications. Medications started in the ICU should have clear indications and plan for duration, cessation, or tapering to prevent unnecessary continuation on transfer or downgrade from the critical care team.

HOSPITAL DISCHARGE AND TRANSITIONS OF CARE

Transitioning from the hospital setting to the nursing home, acute rehabilitation unit or home with primary care can be fraught with difficulty as provider-to-provider handoffs can be inconsistent and patients may not understand their medication regimen. Risk of polypharmacy increases due to difficulties such as a change in formulary between the hospital to the nursing home or outpatient pharmacy and missed or extra doses of a medication depending on medication dose timing on discharge followed by patient transportation and delay in reconciliation at a facility or delay in pharmacy pick up. Reduction in polypharmacy and medication errors can be achieved through four main principles: provider handoffs, medication reconciliation, patient and caregiver education, and pharmacy formulary reconciliation.

Provider Handoffs

Most medication errors occur due to a lack of effective communication between providers during transitions of care.[74] When transitioning from a hospital to an outside facility, the ideal provider-to-provider handoff should be completed within 24 hours of hospital discharge to reduce medication mismanagement. The same guidance applies to patients who are returning home and will resume care with their PCP. These conversations can help providers better understand acute versus maintenance medications to reduce polypharmacy in the long term. Enough medication should be prescribed to bridge until the patient's next primary care follow-up.

Medication Reconciliation

All electronic medical records (EMRs) require a medication reconciliation before discharge, but most recent medication administration and next administration time can be vague. On discharge to another facility, patients should be transported immediately after administration of medication to diminish missed doses or alternatively double dosing if the receiving facility rushes the medication reconciliation to give medications.[75] For patients transitioning home, noting the time of the next medication dose will clarify for patients and caregivers the timing of medication administration. Clinicians should complete the medication reconciliation with the patient, and provide the patient with a printed list of all medications and details regarding any medication changes.

Patient Knowledge

Despite education at the end of hospitalization, less than half of patients can correctly describe their medication regimen on discharge.[76] There are many factors that contribute to this, including length of hospitalization, number of changes from home regimen, and new medications. Of newly prescribed medications, 11% of patients could name the medication, but not the correct dosage or indication; notably, high-risk medications such as oral anticoagulants and opioid analgesics were named correctly approximately 40% of the time.[76] It is important to include patient caregivers into conversations on medication changes so they can reassure and confirm changes to the patient once at home.[77] Clinicians should take special care when changing long-standing medications, as any change in number, shape, or color of a pill can confuse patients when they've become accustomed to a certain regimen.[78] In addition, these changes should be included in the discharge instructions, and instructions for patients to pick up medications from the pharmacy shortly after discharge.[79]

Some additional considerations for reducing polypharmacy after discharge include:

- For short-term medicines, such as completing an antibiotic course, or medications critical to the safety and health of the patient, ensure the patient has the medication in hand before the patient is discharged.
- Be cautious with the use of splitting scored medications or having patients take multiple pills for higher total dosages to save money on medications they already have at home. Complicated medication regimens will cause confusion and create unnecessary risks for patients
- To prevent patients from taking two of the same medications, use discretion when refilling unchanged home medications that patients and caregivers state they have enough of at home.

Pharmacy Formulary Reconciliation

Continuity of pharmaceutical care is beneficial for the patient, especially when patients move between facilities with different formularies. To navigate this transition, consider:

- Document any medication changes made on admission in the paperwork sent with the patient to the receiving facility.

- Send prescriptions to the patient's customary pharmacy to eliminate medication changes due to formulary differences,[80,81] and to ensure unchanged home medications are not filled in duplicate).[79,82]
- Clinicians should communicate with pharmacies as needed to discuss any medication discrepancies or changes to previous medications.[80]

TOOLS TO HELP CLINICIANS REDUCE POLYPHARMACY

There are two primary tools that clinicians use to minimize the risk of polypharmacy in older adults: Beers Criteria from the American Geriatric Society (Beers Criteria)[55] and Screening Tool of Older People's Prescriptions (STOPP) and Screening Tool to Alert to Right Treatment (START).[83] A 3rd decision tool, the PRISCUS list,[84] has been used more broadly in Europe. Beers Criteria are published as a list of medications by class alongside a recommendation; each recommendation has a rationale, a recommendation strength, and an evidence strength. Recommendations range from simply "Avoid" to "Use with caution" with caveats of specific instances that require avoidance or caution. The graphs are easy to use for the experienced or training clinician and could easily be implemented into an EMR as a notation in medication orders. STOPP/START criteria are sorted by body system and guide the provider in decision-making regarding medication prescriptions. When applied at a single time point during hospitalization for acute illness in older adults, STOPP/START significantly improves medication appropriateness and that effect was maintained 6 months post-intervention.[85] When compared head-to-head, PIM prevalence rates on admission between STOPP/START and Beers criteria were similar (77% and 89%, respectively) and considerably higher than the PRISCUS list (42%).[86] On hospital discharge, use of either tool led to PIM prevalence of less than 10% and total number of prescriptions were not statistically different between them.[86]

Limitations of Decision Tools in the Hospital Setting

Hospitals across the country have implemented versions of these decision tools into EMR or pharmacy protocols, including as a hard stop or soft stop/pop-up notification when a medication on the list is ordered on a patient over 65 years. Only 65% of the STOPP/START criteria can be converted to a computerized algorithm.[87] Unfortunately, computer-based algorithms have not had significant uptake by providers or shown efficacy in reducing polypharmacy.[6] Younger providers or trainees may not understand the method behind these decision support tools and may shy away from medications that elicit a warning even if they are medically appropriate. It is important that educators make clear the intent behind these tools which flag PIMs, and help trainees determine in what cases they might be appropriate.

SUMMARY

Polypharmacy in the older adult is an unsafe condition that may cause patients irreversible harm. Hospital-based providers are key to reducing polypharmacy for older adults through their medication reconciliation processes, careful attention to medication use during key clinical scenarios, and strict attention to detail at the time of transitioning patients out of the hospital.

CLINICS CARE POINTS

- As many adverse drug events are dose-related, using the mantra "start low and go slow" for medication dose adjustments may prevent many hospitalizations or in-hospital complications due to adverse drug events.

- A multidisciplinary team approach, including addition of hospital pharmacists in the reconciliation process, improves identification of potential drug-related problems, especially in special populations such as chronic kidney disease.
- Patients should be counseled to wear an alert bracelet, keep an updated and accurate medication list, and ensure familiarity with medications in case of emergencies.
- Patients should be counseled on expected versus concerning side effects that require urgent evaluation and strategies to manage expected side effects of medications prescribed.
- A systematic approach for deprescribing should be taken, including reviewing indications for medications, identifying potentially inappropriate medications, determining whether medications will require tapering or monitoring on modification, and reviewing patient and caregiver preferences.
- Reduction in polypharmacy and medication errors during transitions of care can be achieved through effective provider handoffs, medication reconciliation, patient and caregiver education, and pharmacy formulary reconciliation.
- Tools for the hospital provider include Beers Criteria from the American Geriatric Society and Screening Tool of Older People's Prescriptions and Screening Tool to Alert to Right Treatment and provide decision support to hospital providers to reduce polypharmacy.

DISCLOSURE

The authors have nothing to disclose

REFERENCES

1. Safran DG, Neuman P, Schoen C, et al. Prescription drug coverage and seniors: findings from a 2003 national survey. Health Aff (Millwood) 2005;24(S1). Suppl Web Exclusives:W5-W166.
2. Albert M, McCaig LF, Ashman JJ. Emergency department visits by Persons aged 65 and over: United States, 2009–2010. NCHS data Brief. 2013. Available at: https://www.cdc.gov/nchs/data/databriefs/db130.pdf. Accessed June 21, 2022.
3. Shehab N, Lovegrove MC, Geller AI, et al. US emergency department visits for outpatient Adverse drug events, 2013-2014. JAMA 2016;316(20):2115–25.
4. Oscanoa TJ, Lizaraso F, Carvajal A. Hospital admissions due to adverse drug reactions in the elderly. A meta-analysis. Eur J Clin Pharmacol 2017;73(6):759–70.
5. Trumic E, Pranjic N, Begic L, et al. Idiosyncratic adverse reactions of most frequent drug combinations longterm use among hospitalized patients with polypharmacy. Med Arch 2012;66(4):243–8.
6. O'Mahony D, Gudmundsson A, Soiza RL, et al. Prevention of adverse drug reactions in hospitalized older patients with multi-morbidity and polypharmacy: the SENATOR* randomized controlled clinical trial. Age Ageing 2020;49(4):605–14, published correction appears in Age Ageing. 2021 Nov 10;50(6):e10-e11.
7. Beuscart JB, Pelayo S, Robert L, et al. Medication review and reconciliation in older adults. Eur Geriatr Med 2021;12(3):499–507.
8. Chiarelli MT, Antoniazzi S, Cortesi L, et al. Pharmacist-driven medication recognition/reconciliation in older medical patients. Eur J Intern Med 2021;83:39–44.
9. US Preventive Services Task Force. Vitamin, Mineral, and multivitamin Supplementation to prevent cardiovascular disease and cancer: US preventive services Task force recommendation Statement. JAMA 2022;327(23):2326–33.
10. Hughes CM, McElnay JC, Fleming GF. Benefits and risks of self medication. Drug Saf 2001;24(14):1027–37.

11. Geller AI, Shehab N, Weidle NJ, et al. Emergency department visits for adverse events related to dietary supplements. N Engl J Med 2015;373:1531–40.
12. Pitkälä KH, Suominen MH, Bell JS, et al. Herbal medications and other dietary supplements. A clinical review for physicians caring for older people. Ann Med 2016;48(8):586–602.
13. Awortwe C, Makiwane M, Reuter H, et al. Critical evaluation of causality assessment of herb-drug interactions in patients. Br J Clin Pharmacol 2018;84(4): 679–93.
14. Agency for Healthcare research and Quality. HCUPnet. Healthcare Cost and Utilization Project (HCUP). Available at: www.hcupnet.ahrq.gov/. Accessed June 13, 2022.
15. Hajjar ER, Hanlon JT, Sloane RJ, et al. Unnecessary drug use in frail older people at hospital discharge. J Am Geriatr Soc 2005;53:1518–23.
16. Centers for Medicare & Medicaid services. Chronic conditions among Medicare beneficiaries. Available at: https://www.cms.gov/Research-Statistics-Data-and-Systems/Statistics-Trends-and-Reports/Chronic-Conditions/Chartbook_Charts. html. Accessed June 8. 2022.
17. Bauersachs RM, Herold J. Oral anticoagulation in the elderly and frail. Hamostaseologie 2020;40(1):74–83.
18. Parks AL, Fang MC. Anticoagulation in older adults with multimorbidity. Clin Geriatr Med 2016;32(2):331–46.
19. Budnitz DS, Lovegrove ML, Shehab N, et al. Emergency hospitalizations for adverse drug events in older Americans. N Engl J Med 2011;365:2002–12.
20. Ruff C, Giugliano RP, Braunwald E, et al. Comparison of the efficacy and safety of new oral anticoagulants with warfarin in patients with atrial fibrillation: a meta-analysis of randomised trials. Lancet 2014;383:955–62.
21. Yancy CW, Jessup M, Bozkurt B, et al. 2013 ACCF/AHA guideline for the management of heart failure: executive summary: a report of the American College of Cardiology Foundation/American Heart Association Task Force on practice guidelines. Circulation 2013;128(16):1810–52.
22. Unlu O, Levitan EB, Reshetnyak E, et al. Polypharmacy in older adults hospitalized for heart failure. Circ Heart Fail 2020;13(11):e006977.
23. Sztramko R, Chau V, Wong R. Adverse drug events and associated factors in heart failure therapy among the very elderly. Can Geriatr J 2011;14(4):79–92.
24. Mets T, De Bock V, Praet JP. First-dose hypotension, ACE inhibitors, and heart failure in the elderly. Lancet 1992;339(8807):1487.
25. Haffner CA, Kendall MJ, Struthers AD, et al. Effects of captopril and enalapril on renal function in elderly patients with chronic heart failure. Postgrad Med J 1995; 71(835):287–92.
26. Rao VN, Fudim M, Savarese G, et al. Polypharmacy in heart failure with reduced Ejection fraction: Progress, not problem. Am J Med 2021;134(9):1068–70.
27. Goyal P, Mangal S, Krishnaswami A, et al. Polypharmacy in heart failure: Progress but also problem. Am J Med 2021;134(9):1071–3.
28. Singh D, Agusti A, Anzueto A, et al. Global strategy for the diagnosis, management, and prevention of chronic obstructive Lung disease: the GOLD science committee report 2019. Eur Respir J 2019;53(5):1900164.
29. Putcha N, Wise RA. Medication regimens for managing COPD exacerbations. Respir Care 2018;63(6):773–82.
30. Polański J, Chabowski M, Świątoniowska-Lonc N, et al. Medication compliance in COPD patients. Adv Exp Med Biol 2020;1279:81–91.

31. McCarthy B, Casey D, Devane D, et al. Pulmonary rehabilitation for chronic obstructive pulmonary disease. Cochrane Database Syst Rev 2015;23(2): CD003793.
32. Safka KA, McIvor RA. Non-pharmacological management of chronic obstructive pulmonary disease. Ulster Med J 2015;84(1):13–21.
33. Noor S, Ismail M, Ali Z. Potential drug-drug interactions among pneumonia patients: do these matter in clinical perspectives? BMC Pharmacol Toxicol 2019; 20(1):45.
34. Kennedy KE, Teng C, Patek TM, et al. Hypoglycemia associated with antibiotics Alone and in combination with Sulfonylureas and Meglitinides: an Epidemiologic Surveillance study of the FDA adverse event reporting system (FAERS). Drug Saf 2020;43(4):363–9.
35. Akhtar A, Ahmad Hassali MA, Zainal H, et al. A cross-Sectional assessment of urinary Tract infections among geriatric patients: prevalence, medication regimen complexity, and factors associated with treatment outcomes. Front Public Health 2021;9:657199.
36. Iloanusi S, Mgbere O, Essien EJ. Polypharmacy among COVID-19 patients: a systematic review. J Am Pharm Assoc (2003) 2021;61(5):e14–25.
37. Kimura H, Tanaka K, Saito H, et al. Association of polypharmacy with kidney disease progression in adults with CKD. Clin J Am Soc Nephrol 2021;16(12): 1797–804.
38. Cashion W, McClellan W, Judd S, et al. Polypharmacy and mortality association by chronic kidney disease status: the reasons for Geographic and Racial differences in stroke study. Pharmacol Res Perspect 2021;9(4):e00823.
39. Laville SM, Gras-Champel V, Moragny J, et al. Adverse drug reactions in patients with CKD. Clin J Am Soc Nephrol 2020;15(8):1090–102.
40. Mason NA. Polypharmacy and medication-related complications in the chronic kidney disease patient. Curr Opin Nephrol Hypertens 2011;20(5):492–7.
41. Peron EP, Ogbonna KC, Donohoe KL. Antidiabetic medications and polypharmacy. Clin Geriatr Med 2015;31(1):17–vii.
42. NICE-SUGAR Study Investigators, Finfer S, Chittock DR, et al. Intensive versus conventional glucose control in critically ill patients. N Engl J Med 2009; 360(13):1283–97.
43. Vasilevskis EE, Shah AS, Hollingsworth EK, et al. A patient-centered deprescribing intervention for hospitalized older patients with polypharmacy: rationale and design of the Shed-MEDS randomized controlled trial. BMC Health Serv Res 2019;19(1):165.
44. Petersen AW, Shah AS, Simmons SF, et al. Shed-MEDS: pilot of a patient-centered deprescribing framework reduces medications in hospitalized older adults being transferred to inpatient postacute care. Ther Adv Drug Saf 2018; 9(9):523–33.
45. Thillainadesan J, Gnjidic D, Green S, et al. Impact of deprescribing interventions in older hospitalised patients on prescribing and clinical outcomes: a systematic review of randomised trials. Drugs Aging 2018;35(4):303–19.
46. Elbeddini A, Sawhney M, Tayefehchamani Y, et al. Deprescribing for all: a narrative review identifying inappropriate polypharmacy for all ages in hospital settings. BMJ Open Qual 2021;10(3):e001509.
47. Kaminaga M, Komagamine J, Tatsumi S. The effects of in-hospital deprescribing on potential prescribing omission in hospitalized elderly patients with polypharmacy. Sci Rep 2021;11(1):8898.

48. Counter D, Millar JWT, McLay JS. Hospital readmissions, mortality and potentially inappropriate prescribing: a retrospective study of older adults discharged from hospital. Br J Clin Pharmacol 2018;84(8):1757–63.
49. Barnett SR. Polypharmacy and perioperative medications in the elderly. Anesthesiol Clin 2009;27(3).
50. Sampson EL, Blanchard MR, Jones L, et al. Dementia in the acute hospital: prospective cohort study of prevalence and mortality. Br J Psychiatry 2009;195(1): 61–6, published correction appears in Br J Psychiatry. 2013 Feb;202:156.
51. Mohanty S, Rosenthal RA, Russell MM, et al. Optimal perioperative management of the geriatric patient: a best practices guideline from the American College of surgeons NSQIP and the American geriatrics Society. J Am Coll Surg 2016; 222(5):930–47.
52. Chow WB, Rosenthal RA, Merkow RP, et al. Optimal preoperative assessment of the geriatric surgical patient: a best practices guideline from the American College of surgeons national surgical Quality Improvement Program and the American geriatrics Society. J Am Coll Surg 2012;215(4):453–66.
53. Park HY, Kim S, Sohn HS, et al. The association between polypharmacy and hip fracture in Osteoporotic women: a Nested case-control study in South Korea. Clin Drug Investig 2019;39(1):63–71.
54. Härstedt M, Rogmark C, Sutton R, et al. Polypharmacy and adverse outcomes after hip fracture surgery. J Orthop Surg Res 2016;11(1):151.
55. By the 2019 American Geriatrics Society Beers Criteria® Update Expert Panel. American Geriatrics Society 2019 updated AGS Beers criteria® for potentially inappropriate medication use in older adults. J Am Geriatr Soc 2019;67:674–94.
56. Subramaniam B, Shankar P, Shaefi S, et al. Effect of Intravenous Acetaminophen vs Placebo combined with Propofol or Dexmedetomidine on postoperative delirium among older patients following cardiac surgery: the DEXACET randomized clinical trial. JAMA 2019;321(7):686–96, published correction appears in JAMA. 2019 Jul 16;322(3):276.
57. Connolly KP, Kleinman RS, Stevenson KL, et al. Delirium reduced with Intravenous Acetaminophen in geriatric hip fracture patients. J Am Acad Orthop Surg 2020;28(8):325–31.
58. Johnson AG, Quinn DI, Day RO. Non-steroidal anti-inflammatory drugs. Med J Aust 1995;163(3):155–8.
59. Derry S, Wiffen PJ, Kalso EA, et al. Topical analgesics for acute and chronic pain in adults - an overview of Cochrane Reviews. Cochrane Database Syst Rev 2017; 5(5):CD008609.
60. McGeeney BE. Pharmacological management of neuropathic pain in older adults: an update on peripherally and centrally acting agents. J Pain Symptom Manage 2009;38(2 Suppl):S15–27. https://doi.org/10.1016/j.jpainsymman.2009. 05.003.
61. Brouquet A, Cudennec T, Benoist S, et al. Impaired mobility, ASA status and administration of tramadol are risk factors for postoperative delirium in patients aged 75 years or more after major abdominal surgery. Ann Surg 2010;251(4): 759–65.
62. Fowler RA, Adhikari NK, Bhagwanjee S. Clinical review: critical care in the global context–disparities in burden of illness, access, and economics. Crit Care 2008; 12(5):225.
63. Bell CM, Brener SS, Gunraj N, et al. Association of ICU or hospital admission with unintentional discontinuation of medications for chronic diseases. JAMA 2011; 306(8):840–7.

64. Cullen DJ, Sweitzer BJ, Bates DW, et al. Preventable adverse drug events in hospitalized patients: a comparative study of intensive care and general care units. Crit Care Med 1997;25(8):1289–97.

65. By the 2019 American Geriatrics Society Beers Criteria® Update Expert Panel. American geriatrics Society 2019 updated AGS Beers Criteria® for potentially inappropriate medication Use in older adults. J Am Geriatr Soc 2019;67(4): 674–94.

66. Floroff CK, Slattum PW, Harpe SE, et al. Potentially inappropriate medication use is associated with clinical outcomes in critically ill elderly patients with neurological injury. Neurocrit Care 2014;21(3):526–33.

67. Garpestad E, Devlin JW. Polypharmacy and delirium in critically ill older adults: recognition and prevention. Clin Geriatr Med 2017;33(2):189–203.

68. Devlin JW, Fraser GL, Riker RR. Drug-induced coma and delirium. In: Papadopoulos J, Cooper B, Kane-Gill S, et al, editors. Drug-induced complications in the critically ill patient: a guide for recognition and treatment. Chicago: Society of Critical Care Medicine; 2011. p. 107–16.

69. Pandharipande P, Shintani A, Peterson J, et al. Lorazepam is an independent risk factor for transitioning to delirium in intensive care unit patients. Anesthesiology 2006;104:21–6.

70. Zaal IJ, Devlin JW, Hazelbag M, et al. Benzodiazepine-associated delirium in critically ill adults. Intensive Care Med 2015;41:2130–7.

71. Wolters AE, Zaal IJ, Veldhuijzen DS, et al. Anticholinergic medication use and transition to delirium in critically ill patients: a prospective cohort study. Crit Care Med 2015;43:1846–52.

72. Barr J, Fraser GL, Puntillo K, et al. Clinical practice guidelines for the management of pain, agitation and delirium in adult ICU patients. Crit Care Med 2013; 41:263–306.

73. Devlin JW, Fong JJ, Fraser GL, et al. Delirium assessment in the critically ill. Intensive Care Med 2007;33:929–40.

74. Johnson A, Guirguis E, Grace Y. Preventing medication errors in transitions of care: a patient case approach. J Am Pharm Assoc (2003) 2015;55(2):e264–76.

75. Allison GM, Weigel B, Holcroft C. Does electronic medication reconciliation at hospital discharge decrease prescription medication errors? Int J Health Care Qual Assur 2015;28(6):564–73.

76. Freyer J, Greißing C, Buchal P, et al. Entlassungsmedikation – was weiß der Patient bei Entlassung über seine Arzneimittel? [Discharge medication - what do patients know about their medication on discharge?]. Dtsch Med Wochenschr 2016; 141(15):e150–6. German.

77. Tobiano G, Chaboyer W, Teasdale T, et al. Older patient and family discharge medication communication: a mixed-methods study. J Eval Clin Pract 2021; 27(4):898–906.

78. Uitvlugt EB, Siegert CE, Janssen MJ, et al. Completeness of medication-related information in discharge letters and post-discharge general practitioner overviews. Int J Clin Pharmacol 2015;37(6):1206–12.

79. Kadoyama KL, Noble BN, Izumi S, et al. Frequency and Documentation of medication decisions on discharge from the hospital to Hospice care. J Am Geriatr Soc 2019;67(6):1258–62.

80. Perry TD, Nye AM, Johnson SW. Medication discrepancy rates among Medicaid recipients at hospital discharge. J Am Pharm Assoc (2003) 2017;57(4):488–92.

81. Van Hollebeke M, Talavera-Pons S, Mulliez A, et al. Impact of medication reconciliation at discharge on continuity of patient care in France. Int J Clin Pharm 2016;38(5):1149–56.

82. Welk B, Killin L, Reid JN, et al. Effect of electronic medication reconciliation at the time of hospital discharge on inappropriate medication use in the community: an interrupted time-series analysis. CMAJ Open 2021;9(4):E1105–13.

83. O'Mahony D, O'Sullivan D, Byrne S, et al. STOPP/START criteria for potentially inappropriate prescribing in older people: version 2. Age Ageing 2015;44:213–8.

84. Holt S, Schmiedl S, Thürmann PA. Potentially inappropriate medications in the elderly: the PRISCUS list. Dtsch Arztebl Int 2010;107:543–51.

85. Gallagher PF, O'Connor MN, O'Mahony D. Prevention of potentially inappropriate prescribing for elderly patients: a randomized controlled trial using STOPP/START criteria. Clin Pharmacol Ther 2011;89(6):845–54.

86. de Agustín Sierra L, Rodríguez Salazar J, Jiménez-Muñoz AB, et al. Potentially inappropriate medication in acute hospitalized elderly patients with polypharmacy: an observational study comparing PRISCUS, STOPP, and Beers criteria. Eur J Clin Pharmacol 2021;77(5):757–66, published correction appears in Eur J Clin Pharmacol. 2021 Feb 4.

87. Nauta KJ, Groenhof F, Schuling J, et al. Application of the STOPP/START criteria to a medical record database. Pharmacoepidemiol Drug Saf 2017;26(10):1242–7.

Polypharmacy in the Homebound Population

Erin Atkinson Cook, MD[a], Maria Duenas, MD[b], Patricia Harris, MD, MS[a,*]

KEYWORDS

- Polypharmacy • Homebound • Home health agency • Pharmacist • Team-based
- Deprescribing • Home-based primary care

KEY POINTS

- Homebound elders are at higher risk for polypharmacy than other community-dwelling elders.
- The period after a hospital stay is associated with increased medication use and medication errors, leading to potential harm.
- Team-based care, including hospital-based and community-based pharmacists and home health agencies, can be helpful in addressing polypharmacy in homebound elders.
- The United States health system continues to struggle with caring for the homebound population.

Abbreviations	
Sars-Cov-2	Severe respiratory Syndrome Corona Virus 2
NSAID	nonsteroidal anti-inflammatory drug

BACKGROUND

The number of homebound individuals—those who never or rarely (once a week or less) leave their home—is rising in the United States. In 2011, the estimated number of homebound individuals aged older than 65 years was approximately 1,974,400, or 5.6% of the elderly population.[1] By 2018, that number had risen to 4.5 million, approximately 12.7% of all those aged older than 65 years.[2] The Sars-Cov-2 COVID-19 pandemic more than doubled the share of homebound elders; with an estimated 30% of those aged older than 70 years being defined as homebound, with black non-Hispanic and Hispanic/Latino individuals having twice the risk of being homebound than white individuals.[3]

[a] UCLA Division of Geriatrics, 10945 Le Conte Avenue, Suite 2339, Los Angeles, CA 90095, USA;
[b] UCLA Department of Medicine, Division of Geriatrics, 10945 Le Conte Avenue, Suite 2339, Los Angeles, CA 90095, USA
* Corresponding author.
E-mail address: pfharris@mednet.ucla.edu
Twitter: @PFHMD (P.H.)

Clin Geriatr Med 38 (2022) 685–692
https://doi.org/10.1016/j.cger.2022.05.008
0749-0690/22/© 2022 Elsevier Inc. All rights reserved.

Homebound elders tend to be older than other community-dwelling seniors (average 80 years vs 74 years), women (67.9% vs 53.4%), and nonwhite (34.1% vs 17.6%). They are more 2.8 times more likely to have 5 or more chronic conditions, 3.2 times more likely to have recently been discharged from the hospital, 5 times more likely to report depression, and 4 times more likely to have possible or probable dementia. They are 2.5 times more likely to be dependent in one or more activities of daily living.[1,2]

Given that the homebound population has a high burden of illness, it might be expected that these individuals are at risk for polypharmacy. However, one could postulate that this group sees fewer specialists and are at decreased risk for multiple prescriptions. It seems, however, that the risk for multiple medication use is elevated. In one study of Medicare Advantage Plan participants, 47.9% of homebound individuals took 5 or more prescribed medications as compared with 27.6% of the nonhomebound population.[4] In another study, the median number of medications in a homebound population was 17.[5] Polypharmacy can lead to confusion, errors, medication nonadherence, medication interactions, adverse medical events, higher costs, increased caregiver stress, and a decrease in overall quality of life for the homebound individual.

Studies of polypharmacy in this population vary in their findings but, in general, the homebound elder takes an average of 6 to 9 different prescription medications daily; many of these medications are to be taken more than once a day.[6–8]

The home-care clinician also has the potential to take a more complete medical history—the clinician is often able to take an inventory of all pill containers, to perform a pill count, to see nonprescription products in the home, to combine pill bottles when appropriate, and to assist the patient and caregiver in proper storage and disposal.

The medical community is only beginning to study and report on this special subset of older individuals. One unique study from Japan[9] studied 153 home-care patients in Japan and found that they used an average of 5.9 prescriptions. Furthermore, 69.9% were prescribed potentially inappropriate medications (hypnotics, diuretics, NSAIDs), compared with 31% of outpatients in Japan. Polypharmacy (6 or more medications) was statistically significantly correlated with age, Charlson Comorbidity Index, functional status, nutritional status, insomnia, and insurance type, among others. One factor also associated with polypharmacy was a 2.88 times greater risk for the use of laxatives, indicating another potential adverse effect of the use of multiple medications. The authors' findings also showed a trend toward deprescribing as a patient's condition worsened; deprescribing principles may be followed more frequently in the homebound patient.

Common Conditions Found in the Homebound Population: Potential for Polypharmacy

Completely homebound elders have multiple chronic conditions, which leads of course to an elevated risk of the use of multiple medications and potential adverse reactions. Among the completely homebound, about 80% of individuals have possible or probable dementia, up to 92% have hypertension, 71% have arthritis, 42.5% have cardiovascular disease, 39% have diabetes, and 30% have depression. Other articles discuss these conditions in greater detail.[1,4,10]

As an example, the Medical Home Visit Program at University of California, Los Angeles (UCLA) is responsible for about 220 homebound individuals. These patients are seen an average of 12 times a year, in order to ensure that any health-related condition can be caught early, and the patient can avoid deterioration of her condition. This creates an opportunity for intensive medication management; for example, if a patient is seen soon after initiation of a new medication (eg, duloxetine), the new tremor observed is more clearly related to the new medication, and the clinician can avoid starting a prescribing cascade by eliminating the offending medication rather than starting a medication for tremors. The home-based clinician is also uniquely poised to recognize when a patient is undergoing a decline in health or functional status and can work with the patient and family to begin the process of deprescribing. For example, a patient with dementia who has been taking donepezil, memantine, sertraline, and mirtazapine may no longer be verbal or experience anxiety or insomnia. It likely is time to start to taper these medications, and a trusted home-care clinician can monitor the patient carefully as medications are reduced. Medications to control diabetes can also be monitored and reduced as needed—a patient who is losing weight, for example, may benefit from discontinuation of metformin and may no longer require a replacement, depending on comorbid conditions and life expectancy.

Hospitalization as a Risk Factor for Polypharmacy

Transitions of care are a particularly vulnerable period for older adults and are associated with adverse outcomes.[11–15] A care transition is when an individual moves from one health-care setting to another. Transition from the hospital to home, hospital to the skilled nursing facility (SNF), or the SNF to home are common experiences for the homebound older adult. Care transitions can contribute to polypharmacy and medication errors in the older adult. Medication discrepancies are common in the transition period[16] and often start at the time of admission because intake medication reconciliation is often inaccurate.[17,18] Homebound individuals are not reliable historians for home medications given the high prevalence of cognitive disorders in this population, and inpatient or nursing home providers often rely on inaccurate or incomplete medication lists found in the electronic health record (EHR). Additionally, polypharmacy is exacerbated by duplicate prescriptions or dose changes, adding to the physical pill bottle burden in a patient's home.

Patients often leave the hospital with more medications than they had entering the hospital, and many of these prescriptions are unnecessary. One study at the VA found that 44% of frail hospitalized older adults were discharged with at least one new unnecessary drug.[19] New unnecessary prescriptions on hospital or SNF discharge include stool softeners, proton pump inhibitors, antihypertensives, and therapeutic nutrients or minerals. Older adults with dementia are often newly prescribed antipsychotics secondary to hospital-acquired delirium, and these may not be indicated to continue after discharge.[20] Finally, documentation errors in the discharge summary can also contribute to polypharmacy.[21] Collectively, this can lead to medication misuse, patient or caregiver confusion, adverse drug events, and rehospitalization.

Of all the various care transitions, the transition from hospital to home puts the patient at the greatest risk for adverse events or rehospitalization.[22] Hospitalized patients aged 65 years or older have a 30-day readmission rate of approximately 20%.[23] Medication discrepancies may account for 14% of these readmissions.[16] Medication reconciliation after a care transition can be complex because it requires the health-care provider to review hospital discharge summaries, pharmacy records, the patient's physical supply of medications (including over-the-counter medications and supplements), and a comparison with what the patient is actually doing in their home. A complete medication reconciliation should be performed after every care transition.

The Pharmacists' Role in Reducing Harm from Polypharmacy

Pharmacists have been shown to play a vital role in reducing polypharmacy and 30-day readmissions in geriatric patients after a care transition.[24] [25,26] A 2019 review showed that pharmacist-led home medicine reviews identified a highly significant amount of drug-related problems including drug–drug interactions, serious drug side effects, inappropriate medication use, nonadherence, excessive doses, and usage of expired medications.[26] A retrospective cohort study at UCLA showed that after hospital discharge, a home visit by a community health coach and a medication review by a primary-care based pharmacist can prevent 30-day readmissions in older adults.[27] The health coach would relay all medication-related information collected during the home visit to the pharmacist who in turn would check for discrepancies by reviewing the EHR and discharge summary and communicating with the primary-care physician. The predicted probability of being readmitted within 30 days to the hospital was 10.6% compared with 21.4% in the matched-control group.

Inpatient pharmacists are also important in care transitions, because they can help provide accurate admission medication reconciliation and identify discrepancies in medication dosing.[28] Accurate admission medication reconciliation will ensure a more reliable discharge medication list. An unpublished quality initiative pilot at UCLA assessed how an inpatient clinical pharmacist could improve the care transition to home in geriatric patients hospitalized at an academic medical center in a Geriatric Special Care Unit (GSCU). The pharmacist performed medication reconciliation on admission and discharge, medication counseling before discharge, and phone calls to patients at home after discharge for all patients admitted to the GSCU. Additionally, the pharmacist participated in daily interdisciplinary rounds and reviewed medications daily. The average patient in the GSCU was on 14.7 different medications. Before the pilot, the 30-day readmission rate to the unit was 23% and 20% of these readmissions were medication related. The introduction of the clinical pharmacist reduced the readmission rate to 13% and only 2% of the readmissions were medication related. This substantial decrease in medication-related readmissions supports the role of pharmacists in care transitions and can help reduce the number of medications in a homebound patient.

Community Dwelling Homebound and the Community Pharmacist

Evidence from small trials in developed countries has demonstrated the benefit of using pharmacists in the community to assist with medication management of homebound elders.

In England, for example, community pharmacists are reimbursed to provide what are called Medicine Use Reviews (MUR), a consultation service in which the community pharmacist provides a medication review and advice on medication management. A pilot specifically addressing the homebound population, a domiciliary MUR, or dMUR, targeted those who could not attend a pharmacy MUR and were taking at least 6 medications. The study found a very high rate of inappropriate medication use, from skipping doses to confusion over dosing regimens to using inhalers incorrectly. Although this was a pilot study, the pharmacists involved asserted that about one-third of the time an intervention reduced the probability that the patient would require hospitalization.[29]

A Canadian trial of home-based pharmacist visits resulted in the discovery of a 40% noncompliance rate, a 21% rate of adverse drug reactions, and a smattering of other difficulties with medications, including duplications, inappropriate medication, and therapeutic nonresponse.[30]

A recent meta-analysis of studies of community-based pharmacist interventions showed a decrease in the use of inappropriate medications, especially sedative-hypnotics (risk ratio 1.28; 95% CI [1.20, 1.36] I2 = 0%, $P < .00001$) but did not demonstrate a decrease in the rate of falls or of admissions to the hospital.[31]

In short, there is much to be explored about the potential role of the community pharmacist in managing polypharmacy for homebound elders; the experiences reported in developed countries are preliminary and mixed. Pharmacists have recently taken a more active role in patient health care, and this is another potential source of help for this population.

Benefits of Management of Polypharmacy in the Home and the Potential to Leverage Home Health Nurses

Another potential source to manage polypharmacy may be through home health. Providing home-based primary care allows physicians to actively engage in behaviors that can help reduce polypharmacy of homebound patients. Because many homebound patients often have multiple chronic medical conditions in addition to geriatric syndromes, prescribing must be done with caution. Typically, patients receiving home-based primary care services do not engage with many specialty physicians; therefore, it may be possible for the home-based primary-care team to assume full responsibility of a patient's medication list and engage in judicious and thoughtful prescribing taking into account both medical and functional complexity.

Aside from taking lead as sole prescriber, a clinician can learn more in the place of residence and by performing a medication reconciliation in person, we learn far more than what can be gleaned in a clinic visit or at discharge from a hospital setting. In the home, we can see where medications are stored and ascertain how medications are administered. We are able to see the duplicate or expired bottles and the numerous over-the-counter medications. When we are in the home, we are able to immediately identify and suggest elimination of medications that are unnecessary or potentially harmful. It is also a critical chance to engage in patient and caregiver education around medication safety and proper administration.

Home-based primary-care providers can also benefit from working in alignment with home health nurses who provide medical services in the home to their patients. They could be leveraged to help reduce polypharmacy. An observational study by Champion and colleagues observed the work of home-care nurses engaging in admission visits with homebound patients with particular attention to the medication reconciliation process. They observed that home-care nurse-led medication reconciliation decreased the number of medications after reconciliation in upwards of 91% of patients.[32] This study lends credibility to the notion that home-care nurses can be used in addressing polypharmacy in homebound patients, providing routine medication reconciliation.

A qualitative study by Sun and colleagues aimed to better understand the challenges that home-care nurses face when addressing polypharmacy in homebound patients. The nurses identified ineffective collaboration and communication with other health-care providers and inconsistent medication reconciliation practices between care settings as barriers in addressing polypharmacy.[33] A follow-up feasibility study by Sun and colleagues in 2021 revealed that home-care nurses are very interested in learning about deprescribing and would like to have tools and protocols that they can use in the home environment when they are engaging in medication reconciliations to help reduce polypharmacy.[34] Further research is needed to implement larger scale education of home-care nurses to address polypharmacy through deprescribing principles and ascertain its effectiveness among homebound patients. Additionally, Sun and colleagues qualitative study results highlight the importance of creating effective means of communication between the home health nurses and the home-based primary-care teams, to help in the process of addressing polypharmacy.

Home-Based Medicine as Team-Based Medicine—a Summary

In short, the home-based patients are at high risk for the deleterious effects on health and quality of life due to polypharmacy. The home-care clinician, although uniquely equipped to observe and monitor medication use, continues to struggle with poly-pharmacy and medication interactions. Additionally, the patient's regimen generally changes after a hospital stay, compounding the difficulty in medication management. These patients are frail and ill, and their caregivers (when there is one) are often overwhelmed.[35]

Home-care medicine should be considered team-care medicine.[36] The home-based clinician can approach the hospital team when a patient is admitted, emphasizing the need for careful prescribing and accurate documentation. One can consider enlisting the community pharmacist with medication reviews and potentials for medication interactions.

Many homebound patients also have home health agencies involved in their care. The clinician can contact the home health agency nurse and review the medication regimen with the nurse, in an attempt to reduce errors, improve adherence, and streamline a routine. This takes effort and time, of course, but may help delay the decline in a patient's condition and reduce the risk for admission to the hospital.

Finally, the clinician can consider advocacy to improve the delivery of medical care in the home. As mentioned above, pharmacists in the United Kingdom are able to charge for a home-based medication review.[29] There have been pilot studies of pharmacist involvement in the United States[8] but there has been little change in policy. Clinicians can get involved by means of their professional societies' advocacy groups or can work at the local level (eg, health departments, offices on aging) to improve health services delivery services in their own area.

Home-based medicine, as a modern method of delivering health care across the life span, remains in its research infancy. Future health services research can explore the most efficient methods to guide us in the best use of limited resources to those who consume a high proportion of them. Polypharmacy is as good a place to start as any.

CLINICS CARE POINTS

- Increased involvement of health care providers in the home setting, along with an interprofessional approach to the care of homebound individuals, may result in a reduction in polypharmacy, an improvement in reducing medication burden, and contribute to an improved quality of life for those who are experiencing multiple chronic diseases.
- deprescribe whenever possible.
- engage pharmacists in assisting with drug-drug interactions and side effects.
- actively interact with home health agencies to ensure accurate medication lists and encourage medication adherence.
- perform a follow-up medication review as soon as possible after a hospitalization or emergency department visit.

DISCLOSURE

The authors have nothing to disclose.

REFERENCES

1. Ornstein KA, Leff B, Covinsky KE, et al. Epidemiology of the homebound population in the United States [published correction appears in JAMA Intern Med. 2015. JAMA Intern Med 2015;175(7):1180–6.

2. Ornstein KA, Garrido MM, Bollens-Lund E, et al. Estimation of the incident home-bound population in the us among older medicare beneficiaries, 2012 to 2018. JAMA Intern Med 2020;180(7):1022–5.

3. Ankuda CK, Leff B, Ritchie CS, et al. Association of the COVID-19 pandemic with the prevalence of homebound older adults in the United States, 2011-2020. JAMA Intern Med 2021;181(12):1658–60.

4. Musich S, Wang SS, Hawkins K, et al. Homebound older adults: prevalence, characteristics, health care utilization and quality of care. Geriatr Nurs 2015;36: 445–50.

5. Monzón-Kenneke M, Chiang P, Yao NA, et al. Pharmacist medication review: an integrated team approach to serve home-based primary care patients. PLoS One 2021;16(5):e0252151. Published 2021 May 25.

6. Golden AG, Preston RA, Barnett SD, et al. Inappropriate medication prescribing in homebound older adults. J Am Geriatr Soc 1999;47:948–53.

7. Sharkey JR, Browne B, Ory MG, et al. Patterns of therapeutic prescription medication category use among community-dwelling homebound older adults. Pharmacoepidemiol Drug Saf 2005;14(10):715–23.

8. Williams BR, Lopez S. Reaching the homebound elderly: the prescription intervention and lifelong learning (PILL) program. Home Health Care Serv Q 2005; 24(1–2):61–72.

9. Komiya H, Umegaki H, Asai A, et al. Factors associated with polypharmacy in elderly home-care patients. Geriatr Gerontol Int 2018;18(1):33–41.

10. Qiu WQ, Dean M, Liu T, et al. Physical and mental health of homebound older adults: an overlooked population. J Am Geriatr Soc 2010;58(12):2423–8.

11. Forster AJ, Murff HJ, Peterson JF, et al. The incidence and severity of adverse events affecting patients after discharge from the hospital. Ann Intern Med 2003;138(3):161–7.

12. Moore C, Wisnivesky J, Williams S, et al. Medical errors related to discontinuity of care from an inpatient to an outpatient setting. J Gen Intern Med 2003;18(8): 646–51.

13. Kripalani S, Jackson AT, Schnipper JL, et al. Promoting effective transitions of care at hospital discharge: a review of key issues for hospitalists. J Hosp Med 2007;2(5):314–23.

14. Coleman EA, Boult C. American geriatrics society health care systems committee. improving the quality of transitional care for persons with complex care needs. J Am Geriatr Soc 2003;51(4):556–7.

15. Kripalani S, LeFevre F, Phillips CO, et al. Deficits in communication and information transfer between hospital-based and primary care physicians: implications for patient safety and continuity of care. JAMA 2007;297(8):831–41.

16. Coleman EA, Smith JD, Raha D, et al. Posthospital medication discrepancies: prevalence and contributing factors. Arch Intern Med 2005;165(16):1842–7.

17. Lau HS, Florax C, Porsius AJ, et al. The completeness of medication histories in hospital medical records of patients admitted to general internal medicine wards. Br J Clin Pharmacol 2000;49(6):597–603.

18. Tjia J, Bonner A, Briesacher BA, et al. Medication discrepancies upon hospital to skilled nursing facility transitions. J Gen Intern Med 2009;24(5):630–5.

19. Hajjar ER, Hanlon JT, Sloane RJ, et al. Unnecessary drug use in frail older people at hospital discharge. J Am Geriatr Soc 2005;53(9):1518–23.

20. Fontaine GV, Mortensen W, Guinto KM, et al. Newly initiated in-hospital antipsychotics continued at discharge in non-psychiatric patients. Hosp Pharm 2018; 53(5):308–15.

21. Callen J, McIntosh J, Li J. Accuracy of medication documentation in hospital discharge summaries: a retrospective analysis of medication transcription errors in manual and electronic discharge summaries. Int J Med Inform 2010;79(1): 58–64.

22. Murtaugh CM, Litke A. Transitions through postacute and long-term care settings: patterns of use and outcomes for a national cohort of elders. Med Care 2002; 40(3):227–36.

23. Jencks SF, Williams MV, Coleman EA. Rehospitalizations among patients in the Medicare fee-for-service program [published correction appears in N Engl J Med. 2011 Apr 21;364(16):1582]. N Engl J Med 2009;360(14):1418–28.

24. Pal A, Babbott S, Wilkinson ST. Can the targeted use of a discharge pharmacist significantly decrease 30-day readmissions? Hosp Pharm 2013;48(5):380–8.

25. Kirkham HS, Clark BL, Paynter J, et al. The effect of a collaborative pharmacist-hospital care transition program on the likelihood of 30-day readmission. Am J Health Syst Pharm 2014;71(9):739–45.

26. Gudi SK, Kashyap A, Chhabra M, et al. Impact of pharmacist-led home medicines review services on drug-related problems among the elderly population: a systematic review. Epidemiol Health 2019;41:e2019020.

27. Sorensen A, Grotts JF, Tseng CH, et al. A Collaboration among primary care-based clinical pharmacists and community-based health coaches. J Am Geriatr Soc 2021;69(1):68–76.

28. Beckett RD, Crank CW, Wehmeyer A. Effectiveness and feasibility of pharmacist-led admission medication reconciliation for geriatric patients. J Pharm Pract 2012;25(2):136–41.

29. Latif A, Mandane B, Anderson E, et al. Optimizing medicine use for people who are homebound: an evaluation of a pilot domiciliary Medicine Use Review (dMUR) service in England. Integr Pharm Res Pract 2018;7:33–40. Published 2018 May 4.

30. Papastergiou J, Zervas J, Li W, et al. Home medication reviews by community pharmacists: reaching out to homebound patients. Can Pharm J (Ott) 2013; 146(3):139–42.

31. Christopher CM, Kc B, Blebil A, et al. Clinical and humanistic outcomes of community pharmacy-based healthcare interventions regarding medication use in older adults: a systematic review and meta-analysis. Healthcare (Basel) 2021; 9(11):1577. Published 2021 Nov 18.

32. Champion C, Sockolow PS, Bowles KH, et al. Getting to complete and accurate medication lists during the transition to home health care. J Am Med Dir Assoc 2021;22(5):1003–8.

33. Sun W, Tahsin F, Barakat-Haddad C, et al. Exploration of home care nurse's experiences in deprescribing of medications: a qualitative descriptive study. BMJ Open 2019;9(5):e025606. Published 2019 May 24.

34. Sun W, Tahsin F, Abbass Dick J, et al. Educating homecare nurses about deprescribing of medications to manage polypharmacy for older adults. West J Nurs Res 2021. https://doi.org/10.1177/0193945920982599. 193945920982599.

35. Foust JB, Naylor MD, Boling PA, et al. Opportunities for improving post-hospital home medication management among older adults. Home Health Care Serv Q 2005;24(1–2):101–22.

36. Reckrey JM, Soriano TA, Hernandez CR, et al. The team approach to home-based primary care: restructuring care to meet individual, program, and system needs. J Am Geriatr Soc 2015;63(2):358–64.

Polypharmacy in Hospice and Palliative Care

Angela Yeh, DO[a,b,*], Amy Z. Sun, MD[c,d], Helen Chernicoff, MD[c,d]

KEYWORDS

- Palliative care • Hospice • Time-until-benefit • Goals of care • Treatment target

KEY POINTS

- Four factors that a clinician should consider when deprescribing in patients with limited life expectancy: treatment target, time-until-benefit, prognosis, and goals of care.
- In general, primary prevention medications can potentially be deprescribed in patients with limited life expectancy.
- Deprescribing medications for palliative/hospice patients requires an empathetic, open, and unbiased conversation about their goals of care.

INTRODUCTION

When approaching polypharmacy in the palliative/hospice setting, it is important to distinguish between palliative care and hospice patients even though the approach to deprescribing in these populations may be similar. A common misconception is that palliative care and hospice are the same. Medicare defines hospice patients as those who have a terminal illness with a prognosis of 6 months or less if the disease were to progress on its natural course (ie, focusing on a more comfort-based approach to disease management rather than disease-modifying or life-prolonging treatments). Separately, palliative care patients are those with serious and/or potentially life-limiting illnesses who are still seeking disease-directed therapies and potentially have a prognosis of months to several years. In the palliative care population,

[a] Department of Internal Medicine, Division of Geriatrics, University of California, Los Angeles, 757 Westwood Plaza, Suite 7501, Los Angeles, CA 90095, USA; [b] Department of Internal Medicine, Hospice and Palliative Medicine Program, University of California, Los Angeles, 757 Westwood Plaza, Suite 7501, Los Angeles, CA 90095, USA; [c] Combined Geriatrics and Palliative Care, Department of Internal Medicine, Division of Geriatrics, University of California, Los Angeles, 757 Westwood Plaza, Suite 7501, Los Angeles, CA 90095, USA; [d] Combined Geriatrics and Palliative Care, Department of Internal Medicine, Hospice and Palliative Medicine Program, University of California, Los Angeles, 757 Westwood Plaza, Suite 7501, Los Angeles, CA 90095, USA
* Corresponding author. Department of Internal Medicine, Division of Geriatrics, University of California, Los Angeles, 1328 16th Street, Second Floor Santa Monica, CA 90404, USA.
E-mail address: ayeh@mednet.ucla.edu

Clin Geriatr Med 38 (2022) 693–704
https://doi.org/10.1016/j.cger.2022.05.009
0749-0690/22/© 2022 Elsevier Inc. All rights reserved.

drivers of polypharmacy are present with most of these patients taking medications for long-term conditions, disease-directed medications, and medications for symptom management. There is a risk that as the number of medications and the complexity of medical regimens increase, patients may not prioritize the most essential drugs. One study found that more medications were associated with higher symptom burden and lower quality of life in patients with life-limiting illness.[1] In the authors' experiences, deprescribing typically occurs when the patient transitions from palliative to hospice; however, the process of deprescribing can begin earlier in the palliative patient's course to optimize their quality of life and reduce symptom burden.

The Holmes' model provides a framework to deprescribing medications in patients with limited life expectancy. This model highlights 4 factors for the clinician to consider: treatment target, time-until-benefit, prognosis, and goals of care (GOC). Treatment target refers to whether the medication is being used as primary (to reduce the chances of an illness occurring) or secondary (to slow down the progression of an illness) prevention. In general, primary prevention medications are potential medications to be deprescribed in patients with limited life expectancy. Time-until-benefit for a medication is the time required to obtain a beneficial result, which correlates with the number needed to treat (NNT). In most cases, the NNT increases as the prognosis decreases.[2]

With the treatment target, time-until-benefit, and the prognosis in mind, deprescribing medications for palliative/hospice patients requires an empathetic, open, and unbiased conversation with the individual, and potentially with families, about their treatment preferences (ie, GOC). If primarily seeking symptom relief or potentially maximizing overall functional status in the setting of their serious/life-limiting illness, then medications designed to prevent long-term complications from chronic diseases may no longer be appropriate. Communicating the process of deprescribing to the patient and family is also important in order for them not to feel like they are being abandoned or that clinicians are "giving up." Relating deprescribing of certain medications to their treatment goals and using positive or motivational language such as "optimize," "individualize," "maximize benefit and minimize harm," and "reduce pill burden" rather than negative language such as "quitting" and "stopping" can promote a process of shared decision-making with patients and their families.

The following sections discuss the most common classes of medications to deprescribe in the palliative/hospice settings as well as offer toolkits available.

ANTIPLATELET AND ANTICOAGULANT MEDICATIONS

In palliative settings, primary prevention is typically not indicated; however, antiplatelets/anticoagulants may be indicated for secondary prevention. Factors to be considered that would shift decision-making toward deprescribing include the following:

- *Comorbid disease*: chronic heart failure, atherosclerotic cardiovascular disease, hypertension, liver/renal disease, diabetes, and advanced age increase bleeding propensity.[3]
- *History of major bleed* or *anemia:* correlate with HAS-BLED score for increased risk of bleeding
- *Difficulty swallowing*: dabigatran must be swallowed whole and if crushed can result in excessively high blood levels and toxicity. All antiplatelet/anticoagulants contribute to overall pill burden and should be considered for deprescribing in the setting of dysphagia.
- *Limited life expectancy or life limiting disease* (eg, advanced dementia, heart failure, chronic obstructive pulmonary disease, or malignancy)[3]

- *Not indicated*: secondary prevention with dual antiplatelet therapy is not indicated greater than 12 months after the most recent vascular event.
- *Drug-drug interaction* (eg, warfarin interacting with other medications to potentiate bleeding risk)
- *Drug-disease interaction*: warfarin can cause thyroid dysfunction, and dabigatran can exacerbate dyspepsia. Warfarin, rivaroxaban, and apixaban are highly protein bound and can become toxic among patients with poor nutritional intake and low albumin.
- *Frequent falls*: falls are common among palliative/hospice patients and can lead to major intracranial bleeds in the setting of antiplatelets/anticoagulants.
- *Unacceptable pill burden/monitoring burden*: caregivers may have difficulty administering medications, and patients may have difficulty swallowing them. Patients who dislike needle sticks may want to discontinue monitoring international normalized ratio for warfarin.
- *GOC*: when GOC move toward prioritizing comfort over prolongation of life, the equation shifts toward deprescribing risky medications including antiplatelets/anticoagulants.

Upon transition to hospice, antiplatelets/anticoagulants can be deprescribed when used as primary/secondary prevention. However, when used for symptom relief (eg, deep vein thrombosis), they can be continued.

Antiplatelet/anticoagulant agents can be stopped without tapering. If patients or families are unsure about deprescribing, a time-limited trial of discontinuation or a switch to a potentially less risky medication can be considered. For example, warfarin can be substituted with low-dose aspirin, which does not require monitoring and therefore may be more palatable.[3]

DEMENTIA MEDICATIONS

Dementia medication deprescribing conversations must be conducted carefully because caregivers of patients with advanced dementia may believe that deprescribing is equivalent to withdrawal of care or that the physician is giving up on their loved one. A useful approach to the conversation is to discuss achieving comfort goals while minimizing potential harms of medications. Another helpful approach is to align deprescribing with goals of dementia care, including symptom management. It may also be helpful to involve a pharmacist in dementia medication deprescribing conversations.[3]

Deprescribing decisions about cholinesterase inhibitors and memantine should be made on an individualized basis, in conjunction with the patient and their surrogate decision-maker. In addition to pill burden, life-limiting illness, frailty, and personal preferences, additional factors that shift the balance toward deprescribing include the following:

- *Adverse effects of medication:* cholinesterase inhibitors' side effects include fatigue, bradycardia, hypotension, diarrhea, nausea, vomiting, anorexia, and weight loss. They can also provoke symptomatic bradycardia and syncope, which can lead to fall-related injuries, including hip fractures. Memantine's side effects include confusion, dizziness, headache, agitation, delusion, and hallucination.
- *Lack of response/loss of effectiveness:* for patients who never received noticeable benefit or who did receive initial benefit but are no longer receiving benefit, a trial of deprescribing is indicated.

- *Lack of indication*: memantine has no clear added benefit in combination with anticholinesterases. Memantine is not indicated for vascular dementia, and neither memantine nor anticholinesterases are indicated for frontotemporal dementia.
- *Severe dementia*: although anticholinesterases are efficacious in slowing disease progression for mild to moderate Alzheimer dementia, they are less helpful in advanced dementia or when cognitive or functional impairments are severe.

Antidementia medication deprescribing should be conducted via a trial of discontinuation. The medication dose should be slowly tapered with 4–weeks between successive dose reductions and involve close monitoring of cognition, functional status, behavior, and psychological symptoms throughout the process. It is important that the individual/caregiver has access to contact a clinician if necessary.[4]

When severe symptoms such as agitation, aggression, hallucinations, or altered level of consciousness occur within 1 week of dose reduction, an adverse drug withdrawal event is likely responsible, and the last previous effective dose should be restarted immediately.[4] When cognition or function decreases 2 to 6 weeks after dose reduction, it is most likely that there is reemergence of symptoms that were previously treated by the medication.[4] In this case, dose increase to the last previously effective dose should be considered.[4] When cognition or function decreases more than 3 months after dose reduction, it is most likely that dementia is progressing, and no benefit is likely to occur on return to the last previously effective dose.[4]

LIPID-LOWERING AGENTS

Lipid-lowering agents have little benefit among patients with limited life expectancy and may cause harm due to pill burden, medication interactions, expense, and side effects. Many palliative/hospice patients have anorexia, weight loss, or poor nutrition for which cholesterol lowering no longer makes sense. All lipid-lowering therapies should be considered for deprescribing among palliative patients. No taper is needed.

Ezetimibe is effective at lowering low-density lipoproteins (LDL) and has a low incidence of side effects, but it is a preventive medication, thus should be deprescribed among patients with limited life expectancy. Bile acid sequestrants are associated with severe hypertriglyceridemia and constipation, and constipating medications should be avoided among palliative/hospice patients who are receiving opioids, which are also constipating. PCSK9 inhibitors are powerful LDL-cholesterol–lowering agents; however, they are expensive, must be injected, and are preventive.

Regarding statins, the time-to-benefit for primary prevention of cardiovascular events is estimated to be at least 2.5 years to avoid one major adverse cardiac event for 100 people treated with a statin.[5] Statins have also been found to be ineffective in preventing cardiovascular events and cardiovascular-related death in patients with end-stage renal disease receiving hemodialysis.[6,7] Statins are known for statin-associated muscle symptoms (SAMS). Subjective myalgia with normal creatine kinase has a prevalence of 1% to 5% in randomized controlled trials and 5% to 10% in observational studies.[8,9] Predisposing factors for SAMS in palliative populations include older age, low body mass index, concomitant use of CYP3A4 inhibitors or OATP1B1 inhibitors, and comorbidities (eg, human immunodeficiency virus or renal, liver, or thyroid dysfunction). High-dose statins also modestly increase risk of incident diabetes mellitus.[10,11]

Outcomes of deprescribing statins were studied in a 2015 multicenter clinical trial.[12] Participants were adults with an estimated life expectancy of 1 month to 1 year, who had been receiving statin therapy for at least 3 months for primary or secondary prevention of cardiovascular disease. The 381 participants were randomized: 189 discontinued and 192 continued statin therapy. All were monitored monthly for up to 1 year.

Discontinuation of statins was associated with improved total quality of life, cost savings of $3.37/day, fewer nonstatin medications, and no significant difference for death within 60 days.

TYPE 2 DIABETES MEDICATIONS

In treating type 2 diabetes (DM2), providers typically aim for intensive glycemic control in order to prevent development of known complications such as retinopathy, renal dysfunction, and neuropathy (which are observed after many years of treatment).[13] However, in the setting of limited life expectancy, tight glycemic control results in increased risk of hypoglycemic events. In a Veterans Affairs nursing home study,[14] 38% of hospice patients treated with insulin experienced hypoglycemia (glucose<70 mg/dL) with 18% experiencing a severe episode (glucose<50 mg/dL). From 2006 to 2011, there was an upward trend in emergency room visits for hypoglycemia, the highest rate being among those aged 75 years or older.[15] There are clear threats to quality of life and higher reliance on high acuity care in maintaining strict antihyperglycemic goals. Avoiding hypoglycemia requires knowledge of culprit medications, a patient's daily pattern of caloric intake, and understanding of insulin pharmacology (if applicable).

Non–insulin DM2 medications with hypoglycemia risk include sulfonylureas and meglitinides.

Consider deprescribing in some of the following cases[16,17]:

- Experiencing adverse effects of current medication regimen
- Possible drug-drug interactions that can lead to hyperglycemia (eg, corticosteroids, antipsychotics)
- Those who no longer want (or unable) to administer insulin injections or monitor their glucose frequently enough to continue insulin safely
- Experiencing symptoms of hypoglycemia but not hyperglycemia
- Changes in their disease process, medications, and/or diet that alter glucose levels
- **Table 1**

Treatment goals for hospice/palliative patients include the following:

- Avoid hypoglycemia while minimizing symptoms from sustained hyperglycemia (hyperosmolar hyperglycemic state and diabetic ketoacidosis)
- Minimize burdens: simplify complex regimens, stop HbA1c testing, discontinue sliding scale insulin, reduce fingerstick monitoring as much as possible[20,21]
- **Table 2**

Many patients and families have a difficult time accepting medication liberalization after providers have emphasized the importance of strict monitoring and glycemic control. This may also be a facet of their daily life over which they are still able to maintain control[20] (**Fig. 1**).

ANTIHYPERTENSIVES

Please refer to Chapter 3 for more information. Briefly, through a palliative lens, antihypertensives can be deprescribed in the following situations.[22–24]

- Mild-to-moderate hypertension
- Primary prevention of cardiovascular events (lag time to benefit)
- Management of stable coronary artery disease

Table 1
Individualized type 2 diabetes mellitus treatment targets

Advanced and Relatively Stable Disease	Advanced and Unstable Disease (eg, *Organ Failure or Limited Oral Intake*)	Active Dying Process
Life expectancy of months to year	Life expectancy of < several weeks	Life expectancy of hours to days
• No specific changes recommended • Modify regimen to achieve patient goals if needed • Fasting glucose target: < 200 mg/dL (a1c < 8.5%)	• Recommend decreasing or stopping insulin and sulfonylureas • Fasting glucose target: ~200 mg/dL	• Discontinue all oral and injectable medications

Data from Refs.[3,18,19]

- Strongly consider stopping antihypertensives in patients near the end of life (given expected decreases in blood pressure and high risk of adverse effects such as dizziness, falls, and syncope)

INHALERS

In the United States, 80% of patients with obstructive lung disease experience inhaler use–related errors, with this risk being exponentially greater in end-stage pulmonary disease and older age patients.[25,26] Improper inhaler technique often prevents patients from receiving the optimal and intended benefit from their inhalers. Attempts may be made to prescribe additional agents to manage uncontrolled symptoms that result in increased total exposure from duplicative therapies from the same class (ie, short- and long-acting bronchodilators, inhaled and oral corticosteroids).[27] Another indication to consolidate a regimen is if individuals are experiencing adverse effects[3]:

- Beta2-agonists: anxiety, tremor, tachycardia
- Anticholinergics: dry mouth, urinary retention
- Inhaled corticosteroids: oral thrush, pharyngitis
- **Table 3**

Our treatment goal is to discontinue ineffective regimens and reduce adverse effects but maintain symptom control. Nebulizers tend to more efficiently deliver medications to those with end-stage lung disease compared with metered-dose or dry-powder inhalers. In addition, switching corticosteroids from inhaled to oral may provide palliation of other symptoms such as suppressed appetite, fatigue, inflammatory pain, and decrease acute pulmonary exacerbations.[28] Consider discontinuing other oral nonsteroidal medications (eg, theophylline, salbutamol) if no longer clinically appropriate in end-of-life care or if there is potential duplication in therapeutic intent (ie, montelukast or roflumilast if oral corticosteroid in use).[3] Most complex regimens can be consolidated (while remaining efficacious) to a nebulized short-acting beta2-agonist/anticholinergic + oral corticosteroid (**Fig. 2**).

OSTEOPOROSIS MEDICATIONS

Please refer to Chapter 10 for more information. Antiresorptive treatments can be used in oncology patients for symptomatic relief of bone pain or for hypercalcemia, and the

Table 2
Insulin therapies and appropriate candidacy for continued use

Insulin Type	Example	Dosing Frequency	Candidacy for Continued Use
Rapid-acting Short-acting (Regular)	Insulin lispro Human insulin (Humulin R)	Meal-time injections	Patients with variable or diminishing intake (ie, skipping meals due to nausea/ vomiting or anorexia) Willing to administer or receive frequent injections, may require more support at home
Intermediate-acting (NPH)	Human isophane (Humulin N)	2 injections/d	Glucose historically controlled on rapid or short-acting insulin, with stable intake
Long-acting	Insulin glargine	Once daily injection	Stable intake May cause less hypoglycemia, as there is no significant peak effect
Ultra-long-acting	Insulin degludec		Stable intake Role in hospice patients has not been established
Mixtures	NovoLog Mix 70/30	2 injections/ d (withhold if fasting)	May continue if patient remains stable on a current regimen

Adapted from NHPCO. National Hospice and Palliative Care Organization Hospice Medicine Deprescribing Toolkit 2020. Available at https://www.nhpco.org/resources/publications/; with permission.

oncologist may prescribe the antiresorptive therapy as part of the cancer-directed therapies. Thus, discussion with the oncologist and patient about the benefits of the therapy compared with the risks, cost, and burden of treatment should take place if the patient is noted to be declining clinically or having side effects of the treatment. Most of the antiresorptive treatments can be stopped on hospice, and symptoms can be managed with other medications such as analgesics, anxiolytics, and steroids.

PROTON PUMP INHIBITORS

Proton pump inhibitors (PPIs) are effective and generally safe for symptomatic management of acid-mediated disorders; however, they are also often used for long periods of time without proper indication or actual benefit.[29] PPIs have been associated with increased risk of fractures, pneumonia, enteric infections, vitamin and mineral

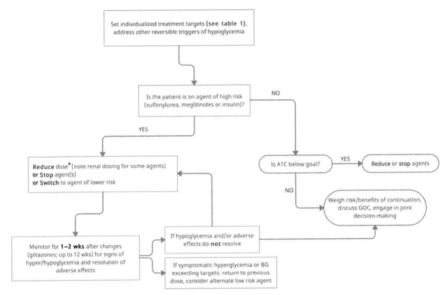

Fig. 1. Deprescribing algorithm for type 2 diabetes medications.

deficiencies, and acute interstitial nephritis. The potential side effects, cost of medication, and polypharmacy associated with long-term use highlights the necessity to consider deprescribing, especially because most of the patients may be able to stop a PPI immediately after the initial course of therapy without experiencing symptoms.[30]

In palliative/hospice patients, quality of life and the patient's values and preferences are important. Some patients find that PPIs improve their symptoms. In these situations, taking low-dose PPIs as needed rather than scheduled can offer a balance of symptom control and reduction of standing polypharmacy.[30] Not all patients are candidates for deprescribing a PPI. Some palliative/hospice patients may have medical reasons to continue a PPI indefinitely or are on medications such as steroids. In these situations, continuing the PPI as long as the patient is able to take the pill may be appropriate.

VITAMINS AND MINERAL SUPPLEMENTS

In palliative/hospice patients, ingestion of supplements (ie, vitamin D and calcium for osteoporosis prevention) may no longer be beneficial depending on the time-until-benefit compared with the overall prognosis. In situations where a patient's prognosis is shorter than the expected time to benefit, there is added pill burden and cost for little to no benefit.[23] Many palliative/hospice patients have anemia of chronic disease that is misdiagnosed as iron deficiency anemia and placed on iron supplementation, which can lead to frequent gastrointestinal GI side effects without any benefit. In most cases in which a patient's prognosis is less than 1 year or if a patient is on hospice, vitamins and mineral supplements can be discontinued.[31]

TOOLKITS

Expert clinical review of medications is the gold standard to deprescribing; however, numerous deprescribing tools have emerged to support clinicians with time-efficient guidance. The following toolkits have been designed and validated for a palliative/hospice population:

Table 3
Potential indications to deprescribe inhaler therapy

Diminished Coordination of Breathing	Inability to coordinate actuation
Decrease in Inspiratory Capacity	Unable to deeply inhaled and hold breath for 5–10 s to allow delivery of medication to site of action
Physical Impairment	Inability to actuate inhaler device due to lack of grip strength or dexterity
Cognitive Impairment	Patients not able to recall proper stepwise procedure
Errors in Inhaler Technique Despite Education	A review of patient's ability to follow and perform directions should be completed at each routine visit; would consider deprescribing if patient is not able to complete tasks despite repetitive education
Development of Adverse Effects	Consolidate duplicative therapies

Adapted from NHPCO. National Hospice and Palliative Care Organization Hospice Medicine Deprescribing Toolkit 2020. Available at https://www.nhpco.org/resources/publications/; with permission.

- *OncPal Deprescribing Guidelines*: OncPal is a validated tool designed for patients with cancer and a prognosis less than 6 months. It was created by systematically reviewing medication classes and examining the literature to support deprescribing. The guideline speaks to several classes of medications, including aspirin, lipid-lowering medications, blood pressure-lowering medications, anti-ulcer medications, oral hypoglycemics, and osteoporosis medications.[32]

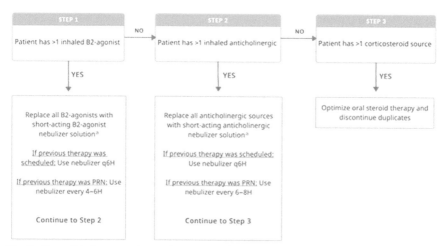

Fig. 2. Consolidating complex regimens in end-stage lung disease. ªCombination ipratroprium/albuterol solution (tradename: DuoNeb) can be used to minimize nebulization time. (*Adapted from* NHPCO. National Hospice and Palliative Care Organization Hospice Medicine Deprescribing Toolkit 2020. Available at https://www.nhpco.org/resources/publications/; with permission.)

- *STOPPFrail*: STOPPFrail was designed to assist physicians with stopping medications or not starting medications in frail older adults with limited life expectancy. The frail, older patient ($\geq$65 years) is defined as having end-stage irreversible pathology, poor 1-year survival prognosis, severe functional impairment or severe cognitive impairment or both, and desiring symptom control as the priority rather than prevention of disease progression. The decision to prescribe/deprescribe medications to the patient should also be influenced by the benefits of the medication outweighing its risks, the challenges of medication administration, the challenges of monitoring medication effects, and difficulty of drug adherence/compliance.[33]
- *NHPCO Deprescribing Toolkit*: The National Hospice and Palliative Care Organization (NHPCO) is the largest membership organization for palliative care and hospice providers in the United States. The NHPCO toolkit is a collection of independent deprescribing guidance documents specific to particular classes of medications and can be accessed online without membership.[3]

SUMMARY

As in the geriatric population, deprescribing is an important consideration for patients with serious illness and/or limited life expectancy in which a "less is more" mindset is often the most appropriate in terms of medical care and the most sensible approach to improving the quality of life of the individual. Goals of medication therapy should be in the context of the patient's goals in the setting of serious, life-limiting illness. If the realistic prognosis for a patient can be measured in terms of months to a few, short years, or even if the clinician would not be surprised if the patient were to pass away in a year, then reconsidering the goals of medication therapy and engaging in an open and compassionate discussion with the patient on their goals of care would be appropriate. When the patient's treatment preferences are elicited and a desire to deprescribe medications/reduce polypharmacy has been reached through shared decision-making, then a stepwise and guided approach to deprescribing with regular follow-ups is recommended as the most optimal way to improve outcomes in palliative care and hospice patients.

CLINICS CARE POINTS

- Primary prevention medications can potentially be deprescribed in patients with limited life expectancy because the NNT of a medication increases as the prognosis decreases.

- Deprescribing medications for palliative/hospice patients requires an empathetic, open, and unbiased conversation about their goals of care.

- Toolkits available for deprescribing in palliative care and hospice patients include OncPal, STOPPFrail, and the NHPCO Deprescribing Toolkit.

- Some hospice patients or families have a strong desire to continue certain medications in spite of the time-until-benefit or pill burden. In these situations, ensuring the patient and family feel cared for and not abandoned is more important than deprescribing a medication as long as there are minimal side effects of that medication.

- For certain medications that are not related to the terminal diagnosis or not prescribed for symptom control, hospice patients may have to pay out of pocket for those medications.

DISCLOSURE

The authors have nothing to disclose.

REFERENCES

1. Schenker Y, Park SY, Jeong K, et al. Associations between polypharmacy, symptom burden, and quality of life in patients with advanced, life-limiting illness. J Gen Intern Med 2019;34(4):559–66.
2. Holmes HM. Rational prescribing for patients with a reduced life expectancy. Clin Pharmacol Ther 2009;85(1):103–7.
3. NHPCO. National Hospice and Palliative Care Organization Hospice Medicine Deprescribing Toolkit. 2020: 1-32.
4. Reeve E, Farrell B, Thompson W, et al. Deprescribing cholinesterase inhibitors and memantine in dementia: guideline summary. Med J Aust 2019;210(4):174–9.
5. Yourman LC, Cenzer MA, Boscardin WJ. Evaluation of time to benefit of statins for the primary prevention of cardiovascular events in adults aged 50 to 75 Years. A meta-analysis. JAMA Intern Med 2021;181(2):179–85.
6. Wanner C, Krane V, Marz W, et al. Atorvastatin in patients with type 2 diabetes mellitus undergoing hemodialysis. N Engl J Med 2005;353:238–48.
7. Fellstrom BC, Jardine AG, Schmieder RE, et al, for the AURORA Study Group. Rosuvastatin and cardiovascular events in patients undergoing hemodialysis. N Engl J Med 2009;360:1395–407.
8. Stroes ES, Thompson PD, Corsini A, et al. Statin-associated muscle symptoms: impact on statin therapy-European atherosclerosis society consensus Panel statement on assessment, aetiology and management. Eur Heart J 2015; 36(17):1012–22.
9. Thompson PD, Panza G, Zaleski A, et al. Statin-associated side effects. J Am Coll Cardiol 2016;67:2395–410.
10. Sattar N, Preiss D, Murray HM, et al. Statins and risk of incident diabetes: a collaborative meta-analysis of randomised statin trials. Lancet 2010;375:735–42.
11. Navarese EP, Buffon A, Andreotti F, et al. Meta-analysis of impact of different types and doses of statins on new-onset diabetes mellitus. Am J Cardiol 2013; 111:1123–30.
12. Kutner JS, Blatchford PJ, Taylor DH Jr, et al. Safety and benefit of discontinuing statin therapy in the setting of advanced, life limiting illness: a randomized clinical trial. JAMA Intern Med 2015;175(5):691–700.
13. Lee SJ, Jacobson MA, Johnston CB. Improving diabetes care for hospice patients. Am J Hosp Palliat Care 2016;33(6):517–9.
14. Petrillo LA, Gan S, Jing B, et al. Hypoglycemia in hospice patients with type 2 diabetes in a national sample of nursing homes. JAMA Intern Med 2018;178(5): 713–5.
15. Wang J, Geiss LS, Williams DE, et al. Trends in emergency department visit rates for hypoglycemia and hyperglycemic crisis among adults with diabetes, United States, 2006-2011. PLoS One 2015;10(8):e0134917.
16. Deprescribing.org. Guidelines and algorithms: antihyperglycemics deprescribing algorithm. 2018: 1-2. Available at: https://deprescribing.org/wp-content/uploads/2018/08/AHG-deprescribing-algorithms-2018-English.pdf. Accessed December 20, 2021.
17. Munshi MN, Florez H, Huang ES, et al. Management of diabetes in long-term care and skilled nursing facilities: a position statement of the American diabetes association. Diabetes Care 2016;39(2):308–18.

18. American Diabetes Association. 12. Older adults: *Standards of medical Care in diabetes-2020*. Diabetes Care 2020;43(Suppl 1):S152–62. https://doi.org/10.2337/dc20-S012.

19. Jeffreys E, Rosielle DA. Fast facts and concepts #258: diabetes management at end-of-life. Reviewed september 2015. Available at: https://www.mypcnow.org/fast-fact/diabetes-management-at-the-end-of-life/. Accessed August 24, 2020.

20. Angelo M, Ruchalski C, Sproge BJ. An approach to diabetes mellitus in hospice and palliative medicine. J Palliat Med 2011;14(1):83–7.

21. Scheufler JM, Prince-Paul M. The diabetic hospice patient: incorporating evidence and medications into goals of care. J Hosp Palliat Nurs 2011;13(6):356–65. Available at: http://journals.lww.com/jhpn/Fulltext/2011/11000/The_Diabetic_Hospice_Patient__Incorporating.3.aspx.

22. Thompson J. Deprescribing in palliative care. Clin Med (Lond) 2019;19(4):311–4.

23. Pasierski T. Modification of cardiovascular pharmacotherapy in palliative care patients with cancer: a narrative review. Pol Arch Intern Med 2017;127(10):687–93.

24. Pasina L, Recchia A, Agosti P, et al. Prevalence of preventive and symptomatic drug treatments in hospice care: an Italian observational study. Am J Hosp Palliat Care 2019;36(3):216–21.

25. Cho-Reyes S, Celli BR, Dembek C, et al. Inhalation technique errors with metered-dose inhalers among patients with obstructive lung diseases: a systematic review and meta-analysis of U.S. Studies. Chronic Obstr Pulm Dis 2019;6(3):267–80.

26. Van Beerendonk I, Mesters I, Mudde AN, et al. Assessment of the inhalation technique in outpatients with asthma or chronic obstructive pulmonary disease using a metered-dose inhaler or dry powder device. J Asthma 1998;35(3):273–9.

27. Russell SJF, Russell REK. Challenges in end-of-life communication in COPD. Breathe 2007;4(2):133–9. Available at: https://breathe.ersjournals.com/content/breathe/4/2/133.full.pdf.

28. Protus B, Kimbrel J, Grauer P. Palliative care consultant: guidelines for effective management of symptoms. 4th edition. Montgomery (AL): HospiScript Services; 2015. p. 225–9.

29. Reimer C. Safety of long-term PPI therapy. Best Pract Res Clin Gastroenterol 2013;27:443–54.

30. Farrell B, Pottie K, Thompson W, et al. Deprescribing proton pump inhibitors: evidence-based clinical practice guideline. Can Fam Physician May 2017;63(5):354–64.

31. Pruskowski J. Fast facts and concepts #321 deprescribing. Palliative care network of Wisconsin. Available at: https://www.mypcnow.org/fast-fact/deprescribing/. Accessed December 20, 2021.

32. Lindsay J, Dooley M, Martin J, et al. The development and evaluation of an oncological palliative care deprescribing guideline: the 'OncPal deprescribing guideline. Support Care Cancer 2015;23(1):71–8.

33. Lavan AH, Gallagher P, Parsons C, et al. STOPPFrail (Screening Tool of Older Persons Prescriptions in Frail adults with limited life expectancy): consensus validation. Age Ageing 2017;46(4):600–7.

Polypharmacy in Oncology

Justin J. Cheng, MD[a],*, Asal M. Azizoddin, PharmD[b],
Michael J. Maranzano, MD[b], Narine Sargsyan, PharmD[b], John Shen, MD[b]

KEYWORDS

- Polypharmacy • Geriatrics • Breast cancer • Colon cancer
- Chronic lymphocytic leukemia • Lung cancer • Prostate cancer

KEY POINTS

- Polypharmacy is common in older adults with malignancies, including breast, colon, lung, and prostate cancer and chronic lymphocytic leukemia.
- Medications prescribed for other comorbidities can interact with systemic therapies for cancer.
- Polypharmacy in older adults with cancer is associated with worse progression-free survival and overall survival in lung and colorectal cancer.
- Pharmacists can play a crucial role in reducing polypharmacy and its deleterious effects on older adults with cancer.

INTRODUCTION

Regular use of at least five medications is known as polypharmacy, which is a common geriatric syndrome.[1] In older adults with cancer, polypharmacy becomes especially relevant as it is associated with multiple adverse outcomes. Polypharmacy is also associated with increased medication errors, poor adherence, pill burden, drug–drug interactions (DDIs), chemotherapy toxicity, suboptimal postoperative outcomes, and potentially negative clinical outcomes.[2–5] Over-the-counter (OTC) agents and natural supplements should also be considered for contributing to DDIs and potentially impacting treatment outcomes.[6] As a result of side effect management secondary to chemotherapy and supportive care medications, additional medications may also be prescribed, which further contributes to polypharmacy. The purpose of this review is to highlight how polypharmacy may impact older adults with common malignancies, such as breast cancer (BC), colon cancer, chronic lymphocytic

[a] Department of Medicine, Wake Forest University School of Medicine, 1 Medical Center Boulevard, Winston-Salem, NC 27101, USA; [b] Department of Medicine, Division of Hematology/Oncology, UCLA David Geffen School of Medicine, 10833 Le Conte Avenue, 60-054, Los Angeles, CA 90095, USA
* Corresponding author.
E-mail address: jjcheng@wakehealth.edu

Clin Geriatr Med 38 (2022) 705–714
https://doi.org/10.1016/j.cger.2022.05.010
0749-0690/22/© 2022 Elsevier Inc. All rights reserved.

leukemia (CLL), prostate cancer, and lung cancer. Strategies to mitigate increased risks associated with polypharmacy are also evaluated.

Breast Cancer

BC is the most common malignancy and the second leading cause of cancer-related deaths in women. The prevalence of BC diagnosis and death increases with age, and these older adults are at higher risk of polypharmacy due to other comorbid conditions managed with medications. The most frequently reported comorbidities in patients with BC are arthritis, hypertension, diabetes, and gastrointestinal disease, which should be considered when reviewing patients' medications.[7]

Many patients are prescribed oral therapies for the management of BC. One retrospective study assessing patients with BC initiated on adjuvant endocrine therapy with either tamoxifen or an aromatase inhibitor (AI)—anastrozole, exemestane, and letrozole—showed the association between polypharmacy and adherence was based on the frequency of medication use, pill burden, and the different medication classes.[4] The adherent women were more likely to have other medications, such as lipid-lowering agents, oral diabetes medications, and antihypertensive, whereas nonadherent women had slightly greater use of anxiolytics, antipsychotics, and antidepressants. Side effect management is also frequent for women who are using AI therapy, and the addition of these medications puts patients at risk for potential harm and complications secondary to polypharmacy.[5]

Certain medications must be carefully monitored for toxicity or decreased effectiveness secondary to DDIs. Tamoxifen is metabolized by CYP3A and CYP2D6 enzymes, and medications inhibiting or inducing these enzymes can either potentiate the effectiveness of tamoxifen, which can result in toxicity, or prevent the drug from reaching therapeutic levels.[8,9] Evidence suggests that some antidepressants, such as selective serotonin reuptake inhibitors and serotonin norepinephrine reuptake inhibitors, can inhibit the metabolism of tamoxifen, potentially resulting in less effective tamoxifen therapy.[10–12] Another example of DDIs in this population is the CDK4/6 inhibitors (palbociclib, ribociclib, and abemaciclib) that are used for the treatment of hormone-receptor positive BC and human epidermal growth factor receptor 2 negative BC. These medications can be impacted by CYP3A4 inducers and inhibitors, which may lead to increased or decreased drug exposure. Therefore, some of these therapies may need to be dose-reduced or alternative options need to be considered to avoid negative outcomes because of the DDIs.[5] Last, heart rate–corrected QT (QTc)-prolonging drugs, such as tamoxifen, 5-fluorouracil, capecitabine, anthracyclines, and 5-HT3-receptor antagonists, are commonly used in BC treatment. It is important to assess the patient's baseline cardiac function before initiating medications that may contribute to QTc prolongation.[5]

Comprehensive medication therapy management should be done periodically to address polypharmacy and reduce potential DDIs. Such consideration warrants the importance of having a pharmacist work closely with different health care providers during a patient's course of treatment, as there are many opportunities for medication interventions to be completed in the setting of polypharmacy and BC.

Chronic Lymphocytic Leukemia

Diseases of the blood and bone marrow are known as hematologic malignancies. One of the most common hematologic malignancies that particularly affects older adults is CLL, a malignant process whereby the bone marrow produces too many mature but dysfunctional lymphocytes. CLL accounts for nearly 40% of leukemia diagnosed in adults with an average age at diagnosis of 70 years. The lifetime risk of getting CLL is about 1 in 175.[13]

To avoid the toxicities that may be associated with cancer-directed therapies, treatment of CLL is often delayed until patients become clinically significant with symptoms such as fatigue, anemia, infections, bulky lymphadenopathy, or "B-symptoms" of night sweats and fevers.[14] Elevated peripheral blood lymphocyte count alone, in the absence of other symptoms, does not warrant treatment. Earlier treatment has not been shown to improve overall survival (OS).

The favored regimen for many older, and often frail, adults is Bruton's tyrosine kinase (BTK) inhibitors, as daily oral targeted therapy with no primary fixed endpoint to the treatment course. There are important adverse events that can occur with these treatments, which factor into the risk for polypharmacy and the prescribing cascade. The first BTK inhibitor approved was ibrutinib,[15] which has been found to have serious adverse effects of cardiac toxicities, increased bleeding risk, rash, diarrhea, and infections. Between 23% and 49% of patients have been reported to discontinue ibrutinib due to adverse events.[16] A newer BTK inhibitor, acalabrutinib, has recently been studied head-to-head with ibrutinib, and this medication has showed lower rates of atrial fibrillation and flutter compared with ibrutinib (9.4% v 16%) and less hypertension (8.6% v 22%), with comparable rates of major bleeding (4.5% v 5.3%).[17] With such outcomes, acalabrutinib is quickly becoming the preferred BTK inhibitor for CLL. Management of atrial fibrillation and flutter associated with BTK inhibitors often involves cardiologists' input and can result in additional medications prescribed for rate or rhythm control and consideration of anticoagulation and may lead to dose reductions or even discontinuation of the BTK inhibitor.

The bleeding risk associated with BTK inhibitors is due to the off-target effect of BTK on platelet aggregation. The risk of major bleeding while on a BTK inhibitor is increased when patients are concurrently on antiplatelet or anticoagulation therapy.[18] Indications for antiplatelet or anticoagulation therapy should be carefully reviewed, and if needed to be continued, patients should be counseled on the risk of bleeding and have close monitoring. Clinicians should also be mindful of the increased risk of bleeding in combinations with OTC medications, including non-steroidal anti-inflammatory drugs (NSAIDs), vitamin E, and fish oil.[15]

BTK inhibitors are known to have multiple DDIs with medications from different drug classes; thus, a careful review of a patient's medication list is warranted throughout the course of treatment. Ibrutinib and acalabrutinib affect CYP3A4 that is also affected by grapefruit, and as such, patients should be advised to avoid this juice. This interaction can increase the BTK inhibitors' blood levels and frequency of adverse effects. Ibrutinib and acalabrutinib should also not be co-administered with proton-pump inhibitors (PPIs) due to decreased absorption, and administration time should be staggered from H2-blockers and other antacids.

An additional consideration for those with hematologic malignancies like CLL is the immunosuppressive effects of some cancer-directed therapies, which has implications for patients' response to vaccines, including the severe acute respiratory syndrome coronavirus 2 (SARS-CoV-2) vaccine. Rituximab and obinutuzumab are commonly used anti-CD20 monoclonal antibody targeting B-cells in diseases like CLL. These antibodies trigger cell death of the cells of the immune system responsible for antibody production, which increases infection risk and decreases response to vaccines for older adults. As such, patients who receive rituximab and obinutuzumab may be unable to mount a sufficient antibody response to vaccines for at least 12 months after.[19] It is important for providers to be aware of these therapeutic effects, so they can best counsel older adults on how to minimize their risks of illness.

Treatments for CLL often involve additional medications for prophylaxis against infectious complications of the disease itself and the cancer-directed therapies.

Patients may be prescribed prophylactic antibacterial, antiviral, or antifungal medications, and depending on the assessed risk, patients may receive targeted prophylaxis against herpes simplex virus, varicella-zoster virus, cytomegalovirus, or *Pneumocystis jirovecii*. It is imperative to note the prophylactic dosing of prescribed antimicrobial, antiviral, and antifungal medications may differ from treatment doses; therefore, careful attention should be paid to the dose and schedule of the medications in addition to monitoring for potential DDIs.

Colorectal Cancer

According to the American Cancer Society, colorectal cancer (CRC) is now the fourth most frequently diagnosed cancer and the second leading cause of cancer death in the United States.[20] Statistically, one in 23 men and one in 25 women will be diagnosed with colon cancer in their lifetime. Although CRC has historically been linked with individuals over the age of 65 years, genetic and growing environmental factors are quickly changing the demographics to include younger individuals. There is a 1% annual increase in CRC incidence in those between 50 and 64 years and a 2% annual increase in those under 50 years. Because CRC shares many risk factors with other chronic conditions, patients frequently must take medications for comorbidities that require chronic treatment.[21] Polypharmacy occurs more commonly in patients with comorbidities, such as hypertension, cardiac insufficiency, acute coronary syndrome, history of myocardial infarction and stroke, atrial fibrillation, chronic obstructive pulmonary disease, diabetes mellitus, depression, chronic pain, and hypothyroidism.[22]

Several studies focus on the impact of certain maintenance medications on CRC treatment outcomes. Giampieri and colleagues succinctly summarize these studies to highlight the effects of these medications on patient with CRC health outcomes.[23] Daily low-dose aspirin inhibits inflammation and platelet-derived signals required for the promotion of specific antitumor immunity.[24] Aspirin also interacts with cisplatin, a chemotherapeutic drug sometimes used in CRC therapies, by enhancing the inhibition of cell proliferation and apoptosis in colon cancer cells.[25] Other classes of medications like antibiotics were associated with an 18% increase in relative risk of cancer and worse progression-free survival (PFS) and OS in patients with metastatic CRC (mCRC).[26] One study found antibiotic use before the start of fluorouracil-based chemotherapy was associated with worse PFS and OS in patients with mCRC.[27] Antidepressants may also play a role in CRC survival. Through a variety of mechanisms, fluoxetine, citalopram, and mirtazapine reduce pro-malignant inflammatory markers found in colon cancer cells.[28–30] Although many common diabetes management medications have shown to increase the risk of different cancers in diabetic patients, metformin has largely stood out as having the opposite effect.[31,32]

Another important impact of polypharmacy on patients with CRC is the DDIs potentially found with drugs used to treat CRC. Patients with CRC are particularly at risk of consequences related to polypharmacy as they often receive multi-chemotherapeutic regimens that require robust symptom management. The number and severity of DDIs are so impactful that patients with CRC taking more than five medications at a time were 72% more likely to experience poorer functional status.[33] Similarly, patients discharged from the hospital after CRC surgery had poorer 5-year OS when prescribed an increased number of medications.[33] Meaningful interventions such as drug-PIN, a personalized data synchronization, and integration network aim to individualize drug therapy for patients with CRC by taking into account current medications and genetic polymorphisms.[33] With a growing personalized approach to health care, pharmacists are relied on more than ever to ensure proper medication therapy that focuses on not just efficacy but also improved quality of life through symptom and DDI management.

Lung Cancer

Lung cancer is the third most common malignancy in the United States, commonly found in older adults—the median age at diagnosis is 71 years and the median age at death is 72 years.[34] Polypharmacy in older adults with lung cancer occurs with commonly used anticancer systemic therapeutics along with supportive care medications. Medications prescribed for other comorbidities can also interact with lung cancer-directed therapies. In patients with early-stage (I–II) lung cancer, there may be drug-chemotherapeutic interactions with potentially inappropriate medications as defined by the Beers criteria, which are guidelines routinely updated by the American Geriatrics Society.[35] Warfarin has an increased anticoagulant effect when combined with common lung cancer chemotherapies, including carboplatin, cisplatin, etoposide, gemcitabine, and paclitaxel. For older adults with early-stage lung cancer, approximately 15% were found to have major interactions between warfarin and these chemotherapeutics in a 12-month period.[36]

Older adults with metastatic non-small cell lung cancer (NSCLC) may receive checkpoint inhibitors (CPIs) as part of their systemic therapy. Receipt of CPI in patients who are frailer can be associated with hospital admissions and risk of death.[37] Older patients who receive medications for other medical conditions experience polypharmacy, which is associated with worse median progression-free and OS in older adults with advanced NSCLC treated with CPI.[37] One contributor is the continuation or initiation of new medications. Among patients with stage 3 or 4 NSCLC nearing the end of life, statin use persisted whereas anti-dementia drugs were newly prescribed.[38] For patients with metastatic NSCLC, deprescribing can lead to a reduced medication burden.

Other systemic agents often used in the treatment of lung cancer include supportive care medications, such as dexamethasone, and chemotherapy, such as platinum-based compounds and pemetrexed. For older adults who receive intravenous chemotherapy for lung cancer, their hospitalization rate is increased among those taking more than five concurrent medications compared with those taking less than five.[39] In a small retrospective case series, dexamethasone was found to have significant interactions with other medications, including antihypertensives. The platinum-based compounds, including carboplatin and cisplatin, and pemetrexed, an antimetabolite, were found to increase the risk for nephrotoxicity when combined with medications, such as antihypertensives and diuretics.[40] Older adults are more likely to have existing renal impairment, and combination regimens, including platinum-based compounds and pemetrexed, can increase the risk for nephrotoxicity.

Older adults are frequently prescribed PPIs and, in some circumstances, without a specific indication. Erlotinib and osimertinib, tyrosine-kinase inhibitors (TKIs) indicated for epidermal growth factor receptor mutated NSCLC,[41,42] have significant interaction with PPIs whereby their absorption is decreased and therefore their efficacy reduced.[43] Among patients with metastatic NSCLC, those who received erlotinib and were on a PPI experienced worse 90-day and 1 year survival.[44] A judicious review of the necessity of PPIs in older adults is paramount but especially in older adults receiving TKIs for advanced lung cancer.

Older adults with lung cancer can experience significant morbidity and mortality outside their primary cancer diagnosis due to polypharmacy. Polypharmacy is not limited only to cancer-directed therapies and may also include DDIs with supportive care medications as well as non-cancer-related comorbidities. A review of the specific indication of each medication is necessary to improve quality of life as well as survival from an oncologic perspective.

Prostate Cancer

Prostate cancer remains the most common non-cutaneous malignancy among men, with more than a quarter million new cases estimated in the United States in 2022.[45] Prostate cancer also heavily affects older men, with the median age at diagnosis of about 67 years, and the median age at death of about 80 years.[46] Management of prostate cancer depends on a multitude of factors, including risk stratification by clinical or pathologic features, as well as staging.[47] Older men may be at risk for more aggressive diseases. A Surveillance Epidemiology and End Results (SEER) database study found that men 75 years or older were more likely to present with metastases than younger men and had a higher risk of death from prostate cancer.[48] In addition, often older men with prostate cancer have a lifetime accumulation of comorbidities, such as cardiovascular disease, and providers must consider the risks, benefits, and potential side effects of systemic therapies for advanced disease.

Androgen deprivation therapy

The first-line therapy for advanced prostate cancer remains androgen deprivation therapy by medical or surgical castration. This can be administered by periodic injections of luteinizing hormone-releasing hormone agonists or antagonists. Alternatively, the first oral gonadotropin-releasing hormone antagonist, relugolix, was approved by the Food and Drug Administration in December 2020. Of note, there are limited pharmacokinetic data to guide potential DDIs for relugolix; however, it has been identified as a sensitive substrate for P-glycoprotein (P-gp) and a weak substrate for CYP3A.[49]

Second-generation hormonal therapies

Abiraterone, enzalutamide, darolutamide, and apalutamide are all oral hormonal therapies approved for use in various settings of locally advanced, metastatic, or castration-resistant prostate cancer.[50] They are all androgen receptor signaling inhibitors with varying levels of pharmacokinetic data, as the latter two are more recently approved.

Abiraterone is a known potent inhibitor of CYP2D6 and CYP2C8 and is metabolized significantly by CYP3A4. Enzalutamide is a potent inducer of CYP3A4 and a moderate inducer of CYP2C9 and CYP2C19.[51–53] In a prospective, observational study of men starting abiraterone or enzalutamide, approximately two-thirds of patients were identified to have potential DDIs with their concurrent medications.[53] More than half of these potential DDI were categorized as D or X risk and with major severity.[53] In general, enzalutamide more frequently yielded a loss of therapeutic effect of a concurrent medication, whereas abiraterone led to potential increased toxicity of a concurrent drug.[53]

Darolutamide is a novel androgen receptor antagonist and has a distinct molecular structure, which may offer a more favorable toxicity profile. Darolutamide is mainly metabolized by CYP3A4. There was no relevant inhibition of CYP enzymes by darolutamide observed in vitro and weak induction of CYP3A4 in vivo.[54] There was also no effect of darolutamide on P-gp substrates.[54] A post hoc analysis of the phase III ARAMIS trial explored potential DDI between darolutamide and common concurrent medications, such as statins, beta-blockers, anticoagulants, and antibiotics. Although the study was limited by small sample size, the overall pharmacokinetic profile of darolutamide was not significantly impacted by commonly administered drugs with similar rates of adverse events.[55]

Cytotoxic chemotherapy

Docetaxel and cabazitaxel are the primary taxane chemotherapeutics used in advanced prostate cancer; both are primarily metabolized by CYP3A4.[51] Although infusions are typically every 3 weeks, the therapies are usually given concurrently with prednisone daily and dexamethasone premedication on the days surrounding infusional treatment to mitigate adverse effects. If toxicities such as nausea, diarrhea, or neutropenia arise, additional supportive agents such as ondansetron, prochlorperazine, loperamide, or filgrastim (or a biosimilar) may be given.

SUMMARY

Polypharmacy in older adults with cancer can directly impact absorption and systemic levels of cancer-directed therapies as well as concurrent medications. Additional supportive care medications prescribed to mitigate effects from cancer treatment further contribute to pill burden and polypharmacy. Deprescribing may improve adherence to medications and potentially impact survival in certain cancers. Older adults frequently have comorbid medical conditions, and prescription medications often interact with cancer-directed therapies. These concomitant medications may affect the efficacy of cancer therapeutics. The potential risks associated with DDIs highlight the importance of integrating pharmacists into the routine care of older adults with cancer. Careful medication reconciliation and comprehensive geriatric assessments can be used to identify polypharmacy and potentially inappropriate medications to minimize DDIs, toxicities, challenges with adherence, and other negative clinical outcomes. Interventions that reduce the impact of polypharmacy can ultimately improve cancer care in older adults, including quality of life and survival.

CLINICS CARE POINTS

- Common medications, such as antidepressants, can directly interfere with the metabolism of adjuvant endocrine therapies, such as aromatase inhibitors and tamoxifen in the treatment of breast cancer.

- Bruton's tyrosine kinase inhibitors (eg, ibrutinib) can increase bleeding risk in older adults with chronic lymphocytic leukemia, especially in patients on antiplatelet or anticoagulant agents.

- Aspirin, some antidepressants, and metformin can have antitumor activity in colorectal cancer, whereas antibiotics before treatment may worsen colorectal cancer outcomes.

- Proton-pump inhibitors can directly interfere with absorption of tyrosine-kinase inhibitors used for epidermal growth factor receptor-mutated non-small cell lung cancer and therefore decrease their efficacy.

- Concurrent medications for comorbidities can lead to a loss of therapeutic effect for second-generation hormonal therapies for prostate cancer.

DISCLOSURE

The authors have no pertinent disclosures.

REFERENCES

1. Halli-Tierney AD, Scarbrough C, Carroll D. Polypharmacy: evaluating risks and deprescribing. Am Fam Physician 2019;100(1):32–8.

2. Domínguez-Alonso JA, Conde-Estévez D, Bosch D, et al. Breast cancer, placing drug interactions in the spotlight: is polypharmacy the cause of everything? Clin Transl Oncol 2021;23(1):65–73.

3. Mohamed MR, Ramsdale E, Loh KP, et al. Associations of polypharmacy and inappropriate medications with adverse outcomes in older adults with cancer: a systematic review and meta-analysis. Oncologist 2020;25(1):e94–108.

4. Calip GS, Xing S, Jun DH, et al. Polypharmacy and adherence to adjuvant endocrine therapy for breast cancer. J Oncol Pract 2017;13(5):e451–62.

5. Farkas AH, Winn A, Pezzin LE, et al. The use and concurrent use of side effect controlling medications among women on aromatase inhibitors. J Womens Health (Larchmt) 2021;30(1):131–6.

6. Wyatt GK, Friedman LL, Given CW, et al. Complementary therapy use among older cancer patients. Cancer Pract 1999;7(3):136–44.

7. Topaloğlu US, Özaslan E. Comorbidity and polypharmacy in patients with breast cancer. Breast Cancer 2020;27(3):477–82.

8. Lim HS, Ju Lee H, Seok Lee K, et al. Clinical implications of CYP2D6 genotypes predictive of tamoxifen pharmacokinetics in metastatic breast cancer. J Clin Oncol 2007;25(25):3837–45.

9. Balducci L, Goetz-Parten D, Steinman MA. Polypharmacy and the management of the older cancer patient. Ann Oncol 2013;24(Suppl 7):vii36–40.

10. Desmarais JE, Looper KJ. Interactions between tamoxifen and antidepressants via cytochrome P450 2D6. J Clin Psychiatry 2009;70(12):1688–97.

11. Singh JC, Lichtman SM. Effect of age on drug metabolism in women with breast cancer. Expert Opin Drug Metab Toxicol 2015;11(5):757–66.

12. Vyas AM, Kogut SJ, Aroke H. Real-world direct health care costs associated with psychotropic polypharmacy among adults with common cancer types in the United States. J Manag Care Spec Pharm 2019;25(5):555–65.

13. Siegel RL, Miller KD, Jemal A. Cancer statistics, 2020. CA Cancer J Clin 2020; 70(1):7–30.

14. Parikh SA, Shanafelt TD. Prognostic factors and risk stratification in chronic lymphocytic leukemia. Semin Oncol 2016;43(2):233–40.

15. Burger JA, Tedeschi A, Barr PM, et al. Ibrutinib as initial therapy for patients with chronic lymphocytic leukemia. N Engl J Med 2015;373(25):2425–37.

16. Estupiñán HY, Berglöf A, Zain R, et al. Comparative analysis of BTK inhibitors and mechanisms underlying adverse effects. Front Cell Dev Biol 2021;9:630942.

17. Byrd JC, Hillmen P, Ghia P, et al. Acalabrutinib versus ibrutinib in previously treated chronic lymphocytic leukemia: results of the first randomized phase III trial. J Clin Oncol 2021;39(31):3441–52.

18. Mock J, Kunk PR, Palkimas S, et al. Risk of major bleeding with ibrutinib. Clin Lymphoma Myeloma Leuk 2018;18(11):755–61.

19. Herishanu Y, Avivi I, Aharon A, et al. Efficacy of the BNT162b2 mRNA COVID-19 vaccine in patients with chronic lymphocytic leukemia. Blood 2021;137(23): 3165–73.

20. American Cancer Society. Cancer facts & figures 2021. Atlanta: American Cancer Society; 2021.

21. Maggiore RJ, Dale W, Gross CP, et al. Polypharmacy and potentially inappropriate medication use in older adults with cancer undergoing chemotherapy: effect on chemotherapy-related toxicity and hospitalization during treatment. J Am Geriatr Soc 2014;62(8):1505–12.

22. Chen LJ, Schöttker B. SIOG2021-0124 - association of polypharmacy with colorectal cancer survival among older patients. J Geriatr Oncol 2021;12(8, Supplement 1):S59.

23. Giampieri R, Cantini L, Giglio E, et al. Impact of polypharmacy for chronic ailments in colon cancer patients: a review focused on drug repurposing. Cancers (Basel) 2020;12(10):2724.

24. Mitrugno A, Sylman JL, Ngo AT, et al. Aspirin therapy reduces the ability of platelets to promote colon and pancreatic cancer cell proliferation: implications for the oncoprotein c-MYC. Am J Physiol Cell Physiol 2017;312(2):C176–89.

25. Jiang W, Yan Y, Chen M, et al. Aspirin enhances the sensitivity of colon cancer cells to cisplatin by abrogating the binding of NF-κB to the COX-2 promoter. Aging (Albany NY) 2020;12(1):611–27.

26. Petrelli F, Ghidini M, Ghidini A, et al. Use of antibiotics and risk of cancer: a systematic review and meta-analysis of observational studies. Cancers (Basel) 2019; 11(8):1174.

27. Abdel-Rahman O, Ghosh S, Walker J. Outcomes of metastatic colorectal cancer patients in relationship to prior and concurrent antibiotics use; individual patient data analysis of three clinical trials. Clin Transl Oncol 2020;22(9):1651–6.

28. Stopper H, Garcia SB, Waaga-Gasser AM, et al. Antidepressant fluoxetine and its potential against colon tumors. World J Gastrointest Oncol 2014;6(1):11–21.

29. Iskar M, Bork P, van Noort V. Discovery and validation of the antimetastatic activity of citalopram in colorectal cancer. Mol Cell Oncol 2015;2(2):e975080.

30. Fang CK, Chen HW, Chiang IT, et al. Mirtazapine inhibits tumor growth via immune response and serotonergic system. PLoS One 2012;7(7):e38886.

31. Chang CH, Lin JW, Wu LC, et al. Oral insulin secretagogues, insulin, and cancer risk in type 2 diabetes mellitus. J Clin Endocrinol Metab 2012;97(7):E1170–5.

32. Pollak MN. Investigating metformin for cancer prevention and treatment: the end of the beginning. Cancer Discov 2012;2(9):778–90.

33. Roberto M, Rossi A, Panebianco M, et al. Drug-Drug interactions and pharmacogenomic evaluation in colorectal cancer patients: the new drug-PIN(®) system comprehensive approach. Pharmaceuticals (Basel) 2021;14(1).

34. SEER cancer stat facts: lung and bronchus cancer. National Cancer Institute. Bethesda, MD. Available at: https://seer.cancer.gov/statfacts/html/lungb.html. Accessed January 24, 2022.

35. Panel. American geriatrics society 2019 updated AGS Beers Criteria® for potentially inappropriate medication use in older adults. J Am Geriatr Soc 2019;67(4): 674–94.

36. Lund JL, Sanoff HK, Peacock Hinton S, et al. Potential medication-related problems in older breast, colon, and lung cancer patients in the United States. Cancer Epidemiol Biomarkers Prev 2018;27(1):41–9.

37. Hakozaki T, Hosomi Y, Shimizu A, et al. Polypharmacy as a prognostic factor in older patients with advanced non-small-cell lung cancer treated with anti-PD-1/PD-L1 antibody-based immunotherapy. J Cancer Res Clin Oncol 2020;146(10): 2659–68.

38. Kim MJ, Duan Z, Zhao H, et al. Anti-dementia and anti-hyperlipidemic medication use at end of life in elderly lung cancer patients: analysis of SEER-Medicare data. J Clin Oncol 2017;35(15).

39. Lu-Yao G, Nightingale G, Nikita N, et al. Relationship between polypharmacy and inpatient hospitalization among older adults with cancer treated with intravenous chemotherapy. J Geriatr Oncol 2020;11(4):579–85.

40. Panchal R. Systemic anticancer therapy (SACT) for lung cancer and its potential for interactions with other medicines. Ecancermedicalscience 2017;11:764.

41. Tsao M-S, Sakurada A, Cutz J-C, et al. Erlotinib in lung cancer — molecular and clinical predictors of outcome. N Engl J Med 2005;353(2):133–44.

42. Soria J-C, Ohe Y, Vansteenkiste J, et al. Osimertinib in untreated EGFR-mutated advanced non–small-cell lung cancer. N Engl J Med 2017;378(2):113–25.

43. Budha NR, Frymoyer A, Smelick GS, et al. Drug absorption interactions between oral targeted anticancer agents and PPIs: is pH-dependent solubility the Achilles heel of targeted therapy? Clin Pharmacol Ther 2012;92(2):203–13.

44. Sharma M, Holmes HM, Mehta HB, et al. The concomitant use of tyrosine kinase inhibitors and proton pump inhibitors: prevalence, predictors, and impact on survival and discontinuation of therapy in older adults with cancer. Cancer 2019; 125(7):1155–62.

45. American Cancer Society. Facts & figures 2022. Atlanta, GA: American Cancer Society; 2022. Accessed.

46. National Cancer Institute. SEER cancer stat facts: prostate cancer. Available at: https://seer.cancer.gov/statfacts/html/prost.html. Accessed February 15, 2022.

47. Tay KJ, Moul JW, Armstrong AJ. Management of prostate cancer in the elderly. Clin Geriatr Med 2016;32(1):113–32.

48. Scosyrev E, Messing EM, Mohile S, et al. Prostate cancer in the elderly: frequency of advanced disease at presentation and disease-specific mortality. Cancer 2012;118(12):3062–70.

49. Yu J, Wang Y, Ragueneau-Majlessi I. Pharmacokinetic drug-drug interactions with drugs approved by the us food and drug administration in 2020: mechanistic understanding and clinical recommendations. Drug Metab Dispos 2022; 50(1):1–7.

50. NCCN Clinical Practice Guidelines in Oncology – Prostate Cancer. Version 1.2022. Accessed.

51. Hebenstreit D, Pichler R, Heidegger I. Drug-drug interactions in prostate cancer treatment. Clin Genitourin Cancer 2020;18(2):e71–82.

52. Del Re M, Fogli S, Derosa L, et al. The role of drug-drug interactions in prostate cancer treatment: focus on abiraterone acetate/prednisone and enzalutamide. Cancer Treat Rev 2017;55:71–82.

53. Vicente-Valor J, Escudero-Vilaplana V, Collado-Borrell R, et al. Potential and real drug interactions in patients treated with abiraterone or enzalutamide in clinical practice. Expert Opin Drug Metab Toxicol 2021;17(12):1467–73.

54. Zurth C, Graudenz K, Denner K, et al. Drug-drug interaction (DDI) of darolutamide with cytochrome P450 (CYP) and P-glycoprotein (P-gp) substrates: results from clinical and in vitro studies. J Clin Oncol 2019;37(7_suppl):297.

55. Shore N, Zurth C, Fricke R, et al. Evaluation of clinically relevant drug-drug interactions and population pharmacokinetics of darolutamide in patients with nonmetastatic castration-resistant prostate cancer: results of pre-specified and post hoc analyses of the phase III ARAMIS trial. Target Oncol 2019;14(5):527–39.

Polypharmacy in Osteoporosis Treatment

Megan McConnell, MD[a],*, Albert Shieh, MD[b,1]

KEYWORDS

- Polypharmacy • Osteoporosis • Fractures • Bisphosphonates • Denosumab
- Teriparatide • Abaloparatide • Romosozumab

KEY POINTS

- In older adults, polypharmacy and osteoporosis frequently occur together.
- Polypharmacy is a risk factor for fractures.
- In patients with polymorbidity and polypharmacy, osteoporosis treatment decisions should be individualized to account for the patient's underlying fracture risk, medical co-morbidities, medication burden, as well as fracture risk reduction profiles, modes of administration, and side effects of treatment options.

Abbreviations	
eGFR	estimated glomerular filtration rate
OR	Odds Ratio
RR	Relative Risk
IRR	Incidence Rate Ratio
HR	Hazard Ratio
SQ	Subcutaneous
PO	by mouth; orally
R/A	Romosozumab/Alendronate arm
A/A	Alendronate/Alendronate arm

CASE PRESENTATION

Ms. S is an 85-year-old woman with a history of hypertension, hyperlipidemia, diabetes mellitus, chronic kidney disease stage 2, dementia, and recent myocardial infarction 6 months ago. She missed her last two appointments and presents to clinic

[a] UCLA Division of Endocrinology, Diabetes, and Hypertension, 10833 Le Conte Avenue, CHS 57-145, Los Angeles, CA 90095, USA; [b] Department of Medicine, University of California, Los Angeles, 10833 Le Conte Avenue, CHS 57-145, Los Angeles, CA 90095, USA
[1] Present address: 10945 Le Cone Avenue, Peter B. Ueberroth Building, Suite 2339, Los Angeles, CA 90095.
* Corresponding author.
E-mail address: MMMcConnell@mednet.ucla.edu

Clin Geriatr Med 38 (2022) 715–726
https://doi.org/10.1016/j.cger.2022.05.011
geriatric.theclinics.com

after sustaining three vertebral compression fractures in the thoracic spine following a ground level fall. Her current medications include lisinopril 40 mg daily, metoprolol succinate 100 mg daily, atorvastatin 80 mg daily, aspirin 81 mg daily, clopidogrel 75 mg daily, metformin 1,000 mg twice daily, empagliflozin 25 mg daily, donepezil 10 mg daily, cholecalciferol 2,000 IU daily, and calcium carbonate 500 mg twice daily. She is vitamin D and calcium replete. The most recent hemoglobin A1c is 9.2%. She previously declined taking injectable diabetes medications. Her eGFR is 70 mL/min. The parathyroid hormone level is within the normal range. Bone densitometry by dual-energy x-ray absorptiometry revealed a lumbar spine bone mineral density T-score of −3.1, total hip T-score of −2.9, and femoral neck T-score of −3.2. The Fracture Risk Assessment Tool-predicted probabilities of major osteoporotic and hip fractures are 34% and 13%, respectively.

INTRODUCTION

In older adults, such as the patient presented above, osteoporosis and polypharmacy frequently occur together. Osteoporosis (decreased bone mass and diminished bone quality leading to increased susceptibility to fractures) disproportionately affects older individuals. Indeed, the incidence of vertebral fractures begins to increase during the sixth decade of life and increases rapidly during the seventh decade.[1] Hip fracture incidence begins to increase during the seventh decade of life and accelerates during the eighth decade.[1]

Similar to osteoporosis, polypharmacy is especially common in older patients. Polypharmacy is defined as the use of multiple medications. Although there is no consensus on the number of medications that constitutes polypharmacy, most studies have used thresholds ranging from ≥5 to ≥10 medications.[2,3] In one analysis of Medicare beneficiaries, ~20% had ≥5 chronic conditions and ~50% were taking ≥5 medications.[4]

Clinical Relevance

Polypharmacy is relevant to the treatment of osteoporosis for two major reasons. First, it is increasingly recognized as a risk factor for hip[5,6] or any fall-related fractures.[7] Second, it informs the selection of pharmacologic treatment of osteoporosis. This is because polypharmacy is associated with worse adherence to osteoporosis treatment,[8] and fracture reduction efficacy wanes with diminished adherence to osteoporosis therapy.[9–13]

The remainder of this article consists of three major components: (1) review of the literature supporting that polypharmacy is a risk factor for fractures; (2) summary of commonly used pharmacologic therapies for osteoporosis and the current recommended approach to osteoporosis treatment; and (3) discussion of how polypharmacy informs the treatment of osteoporosis in the patient presented above.

Polypharmacy as a Risk Factor for Fractures

Polypharmacy is increasingly recognized as a risk factor for fractures. Indeed, data from several analyses have revealed a dose–response relationship between the number of medications used and risk of hip[5,6] or any fall-related fractures.[7]

In a sample of 9312 older adults, identified via the national health registry in Taiwan, Lai and colleagues found that the use of 2 to 4 medications was associated with a 64% greater odds of hip fractures (OR 1.64, confidence interval [CI] 1.47–1.83) than use of ≤1 medication. Moreover, in those using ≥10 medications, odds of hip fracture was ~8-fold greater (OR 8.42, 95% CI 4.73–15.0) than in those using ≤1 medication.[5]

Similar results were reported by Park and colleagues, in an analysis of 5015 South Korean women ≥50 years with osteoporosis. Compared with women taking ≤1 medication, odds of hip fracture was 65% (OR 1.65, 95% CI 1.31–2.08) and 111% (OR 2.11, 95% CI 1.12–3.96) greater in women taking 5 to 9 or ≥10 medications, respectively.[6]

In an even larger analysis of 35,598 older Taiwanese adults also identified through the national health registry, Pan and colleagues examined the relationship between polypharmacy and any fall-related fractures. Use of medication from even one category was associated with a ~30% greater odds of fracture (men: OR 1.31, 95% CI 1.03–1.67; women: OR 1.26, 95% CI 1.05–1.52) versus use of no medication. Among those using medications from ≥4 versus 0 categories, odds of fracture was ~2-fold greater (men: OR 2.16, 95% 1.75–2.68; women: OR 2.23, 95% CI 1.90–2.62).[7]

Polypharmacy may contribute to fractures via several pathways. First, polypharmacy has shown to increase risk of falls. In a systematic review, Fried and colleagues reported that polypharmacy was a risk factor for falls or fall-related outcomes in 12 out of 14 studies rated "good."[14] Along these lines, Dhalwani and colleagues, demonstrated that, in 5213 adults >60 years, use of >5 or >10 drugs versus <1 medication was associated with 21% (IRR 1.21, 95% CI 1.11–1.31) and 50% (IRR 1.50, 95% CI 1.34–1.67) greater risk of incident falls, respectively.[15] Polypharmacy may also be related to fracture by being a risk factor for nonadherence to prescribed anti-osteoporosis therapy,[8] or being a marker of poor overall health and frailty.[4,6] Some medications can also be directly toxic to bone.[16]

Therapeutic Options

This section reviews the anti-fracture efficacy of pharmacologic treatments for osteoporosis as well as the modes of administration and common side effects of these therapies. We focus on the mode of administration and common side effects because these factors warrant consideration, especially when selecting optimal therapy for patients with polymorbidity and polypharmacy.

Overview of pharmacologic treatment

Broadly, there are two classes of medications to treat osteoporosis: antiresorptive (or anti-remodeling) and osteoanabolic drugs. Antiresorptive medications are osteoclast inhibitors. They preserve existing bone mass and increase the degree and homogeneity of bone mineralization by reducing the number of bone remodeling units, decreasing the rate of bone remodeling, and promoting secondary mineralization of bone.[17] Osteoanabolic medications stimulate new bone formation by increasing bone remodeling (with positive remodeling balance) and/or stimulating modeling-based bone formation (laying down new bone outside of the bone remodeling unit apparatus).[17]

Antiresorptive therapy

Table 1 summarizes the anti-fracture efficacy, mode of administration, and common side effects of four bisphosphonates (alendronate, risedronate, zoledronic acid, and ibandronate) and denosumab (a monoclonal antibody that inhibits receptor activator of nuclear factor kappa-B ligand).

Anti-fracture efficacy of antiresorptive therapy. Alendronate,[18,19] risedronate,[20,21] zoledronic acid,[22,23] and denosumab[24,25] are considered the first-line options in most patients because they have "broad-spectrum" fracture reduction efficacy[16,26,27]; they reduce the risk of vertebral, non-vertebral, and hip fractures. Ibandronate reduces vertebral fracture risk but has not been shown to reduce the non-vertebral or hip fracture risk.[28] A recent network meta-analysis, commissioned by the Endocrine

Table 1
Anti-fracture efficacy, mode of administration, and side effects of antiresorptive therapy

Medication	Anti-Fracture Efficacy[a]			Administration	Side Effects[b]
	Vertebral	Non-Vertebral	Hip		
Alendronate	0.57(0.45–0.71)	0.84(0.74–0.94)	0.61(0.42–0.90)	10 mg PO daily 70 mg PO weekly	Upper gastrointestinal irritation
Risedronate	0.61(0.48–0.78)	0.78(0.68–0.89)	0.73(0.58–0.92)	5 mg PO daily 35 mg PO weekly 150 mg PO monthly	
Zoledronic acid	0.38(0.25–0.58)	0.79(0.67–0.94)	0.60(0.45–0.81)	5 mg IV once year	Acute phase reaction (flu-like symptoms, eg, pyrexia and myalgias); rarely, severe bone, joint, and muscle pain
Ibandronate	0.67(0.48–0.93)	1.06(0.83–1.36)	0.62(0.29–1.36)	2.5 mg PO daily 150 mg PO monthly 3 mg IV every 3 mo	PO: the same as for alendronate/risedronate IV: the same as for zoledronic acid
Denosumab	0.32(0.22–0.45)	0.80(0.67–0.96)	0.56(0.35–0.90)	60 mg SQ every 6 mo	Musculoskeletal pain, hypercholesterolemia, cystitis Discontinuation leads to rapid bone loss that is associated with risk of multiple spine fractures

Abbreviation: PO, by mouth; SQ, subcutaneous.

[a] Risk ratios (95% CI) as determined by a network meta-analysis commissioned by the Endocrine Society comparing the effects of the various pharmacologic treatments to placebo.

[b] All listed antiresorptive agents can cause hypocalcemia, but most commonly occurs with denosumab. All listed antiresorptive agents are also associated with rare cases of osteonecrosis of the jaw and atypical femur fractures.

Society,[27] showed that bisphosphonates reduce vertebral, non-vertebral, and hip fracture risk by 33% to 62%, 16% to 21% (excluding ibandronate), and 27% to 40% (excluding ibandronate), respectively.[29] The corresponding reduction in fracture rates for denosumab was 68% (vertebral fractures), 20% (non-vertebral fractures), and 44% (hip fractures).[29]

Mode of administration and common side effects of antiresorptive therapy. Alendronate and risedronate are oral bisphosphonates; alendronate can be taken daily or weekly, whereas risedronate is administered daily, weekly, or monthly.[16] Zoledronic acid is administered intravenously once a year.[16] Ibandronate can be taken orally (daily or monthly) or intravenously every 3 months.[16] Denosumab is a subcutaneous injection administered every 6 months.[16]

Oral bisphosphonates include alendronate, risedronate, and ibandronate (which can also be administered intravenously). Oral bisphosphonates must be taken on an empty stomach with 8 ounces of water (without other food or medications). After ingestion, patients should remain upright for 30 to 60 min to prevent esophageal irritation in case the pill does not clear the esophagus. The most common side effect is upper gastrointestinal irritation. Oral bisphosphonates are contraindicated if the patient has esophageal abnormalities that delay transit of the medication, cannot stay upright for at least 30 minutes, is at high risk of aspiration, or has a creatinine clearance (CrCl) < 30 mL/min (risedronate, ibandronate) or <35 mL/min (alendronate).[16,18–21,27]

Zoledronic acid and ibandronate are administered intravenously annually or every 3 months, respectively. Intravenous (IV) bisphosphonates can cause acute phase reactions, or "flu-like" symptoms, consisting of fever and muscle aches, which last several days. Zoledronic acid can rarely cause severe bone, joint, and muscle pain. Zoledronic acid is contraindicated if the CrCl is < 35 mL/min, or if there is acute kidney injury.[16,22,23,27]

Denosumab is a subcutaneous injection, administered every 6 months. Most common side effects are musculoskeletal pain, hypercholesterolemia, and cystitis.[24,25] Denosumab is contraindicated in patients with hypocalcemia. Discontinuation of denosumab leads to rapid "withdrawal" or "rebound" bone loss that is associated with increased risk of multiple vertebral fractures.[30]

Osteoanabolic therapy

Table 2 summarizes the anti-fracture efficacy, mode of administration, and common side effects of teriparatide, abaloparatide, and romosozumab.

Anti-fracture efficacy of osteoanabolic therapy. Teriparatide and abaloparatide are parathyroid hormone (PTH) and PTH-related protein analogs.[31,32] In the Endocrine Society network meta-analysis, they reduce vertebral fracture risk by 73% (RR 0.27, 95% CI 0.19–0.38) (teriparatide) and 86% (RR 0.14, 95% CI 0.05–0.42) (abaloparatide) and non-vertebral fracture risk by 38% (RR 0.62 95% CI 0.47–0.80) (teriparatide) and 49% (RR 0.51, 95% CI 0.29–0.87) (abaloparatide).[29] There were trends toward hip fracture reductions for both medications, but these did not reach statistical significance (note that the parent teriparatide and abaloparatide studies had very few hip fractures and were underpowered for this endpoint).[29]

Romosozumab is a monoclonal antibody that inhibits sclerostin. Although commonly considered an osteoanabolic agent, it both increases bone formation and decreases bone resorption.[33,34] The Endocrine Society network meta-analysis showed that romosozumab reduces vertebral, non-vertebral, and hip fracture risk by 67% (RR 0.33, 95% CI 0.22–0.49), 33% (RR 0.67, 95% CI 0.53–0.86), and 56% (RR 0.44, 95% CI 0.24–0.79), respectively.[29]

Table 2
Anti-fracture efficacy, mode of administration, and side effects of osteoanabolic therapy

Medication	Anti-Fracture Efficacy[a]			Administration	Side Effects
	Vertebral	Non-Vertebral	Hip		
Teriparatide	0.27(0.19–0.38)	0.62(0.47–0.80)	0.64(0.25–1.68)	20 µg SQ daily	Dizziness, nausea, muscle cramps, hypercalcemia (less
Abaloparatide	0.14(0.05–0.42)	0.51(0.29–0.87)	0.24(0.01–4.84)	80 µg SQ daily	with abaloparatide)
					Note that FDA black box warning regarding
					osteosarcoma removed
Romosozumab	0.33(0.22–0.49)	0.67(0.53–0.86)	0.44(0.24–0.79)	210 mg SQ monthly	Injection site reaction, hypocalcemia
					Rarely, osteonecrosis of the jaw, atypical femur fracture
					Note that FDA black box warning regarding major
					adverse cardiovascular events (use not recommended
					if MI or stroke within last 12 mo)

[a] Risk ratios as determined by a network meta-analysis commissioned by the Endocrine Society comparing the effects of the various pharmacologic treatments to placebo. Effect sizes presented as risk ratios (95% CI).

Mode of administration and common side effects of osteoanabolic therapy. Both teriparatide and abaloparatide are daily injections for up to 2 years.[31,32] Teriparatide is associated with dizziness and leg cramps, whereas abaloparatide is associated with nausea, postural hypotension, dizziness, headache, and palpitations.[27,31] Both agents can cause hypercalcemia, although abaloparatide is considered less calcium mobilizing than teriparatide.[27,32] Both drugs previously carried Food and Drug Administration (FDA) black box warnings about a dose–response relationship between these agents and osteosarcoma in rats; however, these warnings have been removed.

Romosozumab is a monthly injection given for a total of 12 months.[33,35] The most common side effect is injection site reaction.[33] The FDA issued a black box warning that romosozumab may increase the risk of myocardial infarction (MI), stroke, and cardiovascular death; accordingly, it is not recommended for use in patients who have had an MI or stroke in the last year.[27] This warning arises from the finding that in one of the two phase 3 romosozumab trials, major adverse cardiovascular events were more common in the romosozumab versus control group.[34] However, the increased risk did not persist and was small, raising the question of whether there is truly a causal relationship between romosozumab and major adverse cardiovascular events.[36]

Selection of pharmacologic therapy. In 2017, the American College of Physicians published clinical practice guidelines recommending that all patients with osteoporosis or osteopenia with high fracture risk initiate pharmacologic treatment with an antiresorptive agent with broad-spectrum fracture reduction efficacy (alendronate, risedronate, zoledronic acid, or denosumab).[26] Since 2017, several head-to-head comparisons of osteoanabolics versus first-line oral bisphosphonates have shown that in very high risk patients, osteoanabolic therapy provides maximal protection against subsequent fractures.[34,37] This led to the concept of risk stratification in newer clinical practice guidelines published by the Endocrine Society in 2019[27] and the American Association of Clinical Endocrinology (AACE) in 2020.[16]

Evidence supporting greater fracture risk reduction with osteoanabolic therapy in very high risk patients was reported by Effects of Teriparatide and Risedronate on New Fractures in Postmenopausal Women with Severe Osteoporosis (VERO)[37] and the Active-Controlled Fracture Study in Postmenopausal Women with Osteoporosis at High Risk (ARCH)[34] trials. The VERO trial compared teriparatide versus risedronate for 2 years in 1360 postmenopausal women (mean age 72 years). Of note, 100% of study participants had previously sustained a prior vertebral fracture, and 43% a prior non-vertebral fracture. In these women, teriparatide reduced new vertebral and new clinical (clinical vertebral plus non-vertebral) fractures 56% (RR 0.44, 95% CI 0.29–0.68) and 52% (HR 0.48, 95% CI 0.32–0.74) more than risedronate, respectively.[37] The ARCH study compared romosozumab for 1 year followed by 2 years of alendronate (R/A arm) versus alendronate (A/A arm) for 3 years in 4093 postmenopausal women (mean age 74.3 years). Nearly, all (96%) participants previously sustained a vertebral fracture, and 37% a non-vertebral fracture. After 24 months, risk of vertebral, non-vertebral, and hip fractures was 48% (RR = 0.52, 95% CI 0.40–0.66), 19% (HR = 0.81, 95% CI 0.66–0.99), and 38% (HR 0.62, 95% CI 0.42–0.92) lower in the R/A versus A/A group.[34]

The Endocrine Society and AACE algorithms for fracture risk stratification are summarized in **Fig. 1**. Broadly, there are three major criteria to consider: bone mineral density (BMD), fracture history, and fracture probability (in the United States, the Fracture Risk Assessment Tool [FRAX] is commonly used).[16,27] Other considerations can include fracture within the last 12 months, BMD T-score < -3.0, and very high fracture probability as estimated by FRAX.[16] Based on these factors, patients are categorized into four different risk strata:

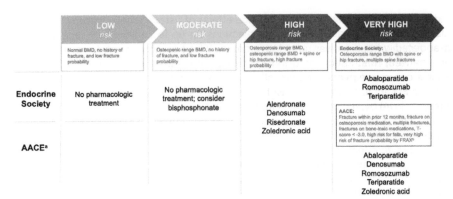

Fig. 1. Approach to fracture risk stratification and pharmacologic treatment of osteoporosis. AACE, American Association of Clinical Endocrinology. [a]FRAX predicted probabilities of major osteoporotic or hip fracture >30% or >4.5%, respectively.

- Low risk: These patients have normal BMD, no history of fracture, and low fracture probability. They do not require pharmacologic therapy.[27]
- Moderate risk: These patients have osteopenic-range BMD, no history of fracture, and low fracture probability. Most of the moderate risk patients do not require pharmacologic treatment, but bisphosphonate therapy can be considered on an individual basis.[27]
- High risk: These patients have osteoporosis-range BMD, osteopenic-range BMD with a hip or spine fracture, or osteopenic-range BMD with high fracture probability. These patients are candidates for pharmacologic treatment with first-line antiresorptive including alendronate, risedronate, zoledronic acid, or denosumab.[16,26,27]
- Very high risk: These patients are similar to the VERO and ARCH study participants who benefited more from osteoanabolic therapy. The Endocrine Society defines very high risk as osteoporosis range BMD with a hip or spine fracture, or multiple spine fractures regardless of BMD. AACE additionally considers patients with a fracture within the preceding 12 months, fractures on bone-toxic medications, BMD T-score < −3.0, and FRAX-predicted probabilities of major osteoporotic or hip fractures >30% or 4.5%, respectively, as very high risk. Very high risk patients are candidates for osteoanabolic therapy, that is, teriparatide, abaloparatide, and romosozumab. Alternatively, AACE also recommends denosumab or zoledronic acid in these patients.[16,27]

DISCUSSION
Polypharmacy as a Risk Factor for Fractures

In the clinical case study presented above, the patient's polymorbidity and polypharmacy are risk factors for fractures. Diabetes is associated with an over 30% greater risk of hip fracture.[38] Diabetic neuropathy[39] and use of insulin[40] are risk factors for falls. Efforts to optimize glycemic control (while minimizing hypoglycemia) and ensure that the patient is not orthostatic could mitigate the impact of these risk factors.

Selection of Optimal Pharmacologic Therapy

The patient is considered very high risk for subsequent fracture by both Endocrine Society and AACE criteria (osteoporosis range BMD with multiple spine fractures, fracture within the last 12 months, BMD T-score < −3.0, and FRAX-predicted probabilities of major osteoporotic and hip fractures exceeding 30% and 4.5%).[16,27]

Based on her very high fracture risk categorization, an osteoanabolic agent would afford the greatest protection against subsequent fractures. Moreover, because she is at very high risk for vertebral, non-vertebral, and hip fractures, an osteoanabolic with proven broad-spectrum anti-fracture efficacy would be preferred. Thus, from a bone-focused perspective, romosozumab would be the best option for this patient; it reduces vertebral, non-vertebral, and hip fractures more than a first-line oral bisphosphonate.[34] However, romosozumab is contraindicated in this patient with a recent MI.[16,27]

This leaves teriparatide or abaloparatide as alternative osteoanabolics. Although teriparatide reduces vertebral and all clinical (clinical vertebral plus non-vertebral) fractures more than risedronate,[37] it is uncertain whether teriparatide or abaloparatide protects against hip fractures. The Endocrine Society network meta-analysis did not reveal significant hip fracture reduction with teriparatide or abaloparatide versus placebo,[29] but a different meta-analysis by Diez-Perez found a 56% reduction in hip fractures compared with controls.[41] Teriparatide and abaloparatide also increase areal and volumetric BMD at the hip, increase estimated hip strength, and reduce non-vertebral fractures (an endpoint that includes hip fractures).[32,42] Finally, this patient recently sustained multiple vertebral fractures, and VERO demonstrated that teriparatide is clearly better at preventing vertebral fractures than a first-line oral bisphosphonate.[37] Based on these considerations, using teriparatide or abaloparatide could be reasonable. However, in an older patient with polypharmacy, it is important to consider whether a daily injection is practical.

Efficacy of pharmacologic treatment depends on both treatment efficacy and adherence to therapy.[9–13] Poor adherence or resistance to osteoporosis therapies is common[9–12] and typically occurs within the first year of treatment, when patients are at the highest risk for fracture.[43] Among Medicare beneficiaries, 45.2% of patients discontinued osteoporosis treatment within 12 months.[13] Causes of poor adherence include drug-related side effects, patient fear of drug side effects, cognitive dysfunction, patient's lack of awareness of severity of osteoporosis and treatment benefit, insufficient motivation to continue treatment, and cost of medications.[13,44]

Although the patient in this case study would benefit from osteoanabolic therapy, romosozumab is contraindicated because of her recent MI, and the patient would likely be non-adherent to a daily injection such as teriparatide or abaloparatide. AACE also recommends zoledronic acid or denosumab as potential options in very high-risk patients.[16] Both have similar fracture risk reduction efficacy.[29] One advantage of zoledronic acid is its long duration of action.[45–47] In contrast, missing doses of, or discontinuing, denosumab can lead to rapid bone loss and multiple vertebral fractures[30] (a concern given the patient's history of missing appointments). In aggregate, zoledronic acid may represent the optimal combination of protection against fracture and feasibility in this patient with polypharmacy.

SUMMARY

Polypharmacy and osteoporosis frequently occur together in older adults. Polypharmacy is a risk factor for fractures. Osteoporosis treatment decisions should be individualized to the patient and account for limitations to adherence posed by polypharmacy.

CLINICS CARE POINTS

- Polypharmacy is a risk for fall-related fractures, hip fractures, and poor adherence to anti-osteoporosis medications.

- Perform risk stratification to determine a patient's risk of fracture. If a patient is very high risk, consider osteoanabolic agents (abaloparatide, teriparatide, or romosozumab).
- Osteoporosis treatment decisions should be individualized and account for a patient's medical comorbidities, medication burden, and preferred route of medication administration.

DISCLOSURE

The authors have nothing to disclose.

REFERENCES

1. Harvey NC, Curtis EM, Dennison EM, et al. The epidemiology of osteoporotic fractures. In: Primer on the metabolic bone diseases and disorders of mineral metabolism. 2018. p. 398–404.
2. Fulton MM, Riley Allen E. Polypharmacy in the elderly: a literature review. J Am Acad Nurse Pract 2005;17(4):123–32.
3. Mortazavi SS, Shati M, Keshtkar A, et al. Defining polypharmacy in the elderly: a systematic review protocol. BMJ Open 2016;6(3):e010989.
4. Tinetti ME, Bogardus ST, Agostini JV. Potential pitfalls of disease-specific guidelines for patients with multiple conditions. N Engl J Med 2004;351(27):2870–4.
5. Lai SW, Liao KF, Liao CC, et al. Polypharmacy correlates with increased risk for hip fracture in the elderly: a population-based study. Medicine (Baltimore) 2010;89(5):295–9.
6. Park H-Y, Kim S, Sohn HS, et al. The association between polypharmacy and hip fracture in osteoporotic women: a nested case–control study in South Korea. Clin Drug Invest 2019;39(1):63–71.
7. Pan HH, Li CY, Chen TJ, et al. Association of polypharmacy with fall-related fractures in older Taiwanese people: age- and gender-specific analyses. BMJ Open 2014;4(3):e004428.
8. Yeam CT, Chia S, Tan HCC, et al. A systematic review of factors affecting medication adherence among patients with osteoporosis. Osteoporos Int 2018;29(12):2623–37.
9. Siris ES, Selby PL, Saag KG, et al. Impact of osteoporosis treatment adherence on fracture rates in North America and Europe. Am J Med 2009;122(2 Suppl):S3–13.
10. Penning-van Beest FJ, Erkens JA, Olson M, et al. Loss of treatment benefit due to low compliance with bisphosphonate therapy. Osteoporos Int 2008;19(4):511–7.
11. Weycker D, Macarios D, Edelsberg J, et al. Compliance with osteoporosis drug therapy and risk of fracture. Osteoporos Int 2007;18(3):271–7.
12. Yu S, Burge RT, Foster SA, et al. The impact of teriparatide adherence and persistence on fracture outcomes. Osteoporos Int 2012;23(3):1103–13.
13. Solomon DH, Avorn J, Katz JN, et al. Compliance with osteoporosis medications. Arch Intern Med 2005;165(20):2414–9.
14. Fried TR, O'Leary J, Towle V, et al. Health outcomes associated with polypharmacy in community-dwelling older adults: a systematic review. J Am Geriatr Soc 2014;62(12):2261–72.
15. Dhalwani NN, Fahami R, Sathanapally H, et al. Association between polypharmacy and falls in older adults: a longitudinal study from England. BMJ Open 2017;7(10):e016358.

16. Camacho PM, Petak SM, Binkley N, et al. American association of clinical endocrinologists/American college of endocrinology clinical practice guidelines for the diagnosis and treatment of postmenopausal osteoporosis- 2020 update executive summary. Endocr Pract 2020;26(5):564–70.

17. Compston JE, McClung MR, Leslie WD. Osteoporosis. Lancet 2019;393(10169): 364–76.

18. Cummings SR, Black DM, Thompson DE, et al. Effect of alendronate on risk of fracture in women with low bone density but without vertebral fractures: results from the Fracture Intervention Trial. JAMA 1998;280(24):2077–82.

19. Black DM, Cummings SR, Karpf DB, et al. Randomised trial of effect of alendronate on risk of fracture in women with existing vertebral fractures. Fracture Intervention Trial Research Group. Lancet 1996;348(9041):1535–41.

20. Harris ST, Watts NB, Genant HK, et al. Effects of risedronate treatment on vertebral and nonvertebral fractures in women with postmenopausal osteoporosis: a randomized controlled trial. Vertebral Efficacy with Risedronate Therapy (VERT) Study Group. JAMA 1999;282(14):1344–52.

21. McClung MR, Geusens P, Miller PD, et al. Effect of risedronate on the risk of hip fracture in elderly women. N Engl J Med 2001;344(5):333–40.

22. Black DM, Delmas PD, Eastell R, et al. Once-yearly zoledronic acid for treatment of postmenopausal osteoporosis. N Engl J Med 2007;356(18):1809–22.

23. Lyles KW, Colón-Emeric CS, Magaziner JS, et al. Zoledronic acid and clinical fractures and mortality after hip fracture. N Engl J Med 2007;357(18):1799–809.

24. Cummings SR, San Martin J, McClung MR, et al. Denosumab for prevention of fractures in postmenopausal women with osteoporosis. N Engl J Med 2009; 361(8):756–65.

25. Bone HG, Wagman RB, Brandi ML, et al. 10 years of denosumab treatment in postmenopausal women with osteoporosis: results from the phase 3 randomised FREEDOM trial and open-label extension. Lancet Diabetes Endocrinol 2017;5(7): 513–23.

26. Qaseem A, Forciea MA, McLean RM, et al. Treatment of low bone density or osteoporosis to prevent fractures in men and women: a clinical practice guideline update from the american college of physicians. Ann Intern Med 2017;166(11): 818–39.

27. Eastell R, Rosen CJ, Black DM, et al. Pharmacological management of osteoporosis in postmenopausal women: an endocrine society* clinical practice guideline. J Clin Endocrinol Metab 2019;104(5):1595–622.

28. Chesnut CH 3rd, Skag A, Christiansen C, et al. Effects of oral ibandronate administered daily or intermittently on fracture risk in postmenopausal osteoporosis. J Bone Miner Res 2004;19(8):1241–9.

29. Barrionuevo P, Kapoor E, Asi N, et al. Efficacy of pharmacological therapies for the prevention of fractures in postmenopausal women: a network meta-analysis. J Clin Endocrinol Metab 2019;104(5):1623–30.

30. Cummings SR, Ferrari S, Eastell R, et al. Vertebral fractures after discontinuation of denosumab: a post hoc analysis of the randomized placebo-controlled FREEDOM trial and its extension. J Bone Miner Res 2018;33(2):190–8.

31. Neer RM, Arnaud CD, Zanchetta JR, et al. Effect of parathyroid hormone (1-34) on fractures and bone mineral density in postmenopausal women with osteoporosis. N Engl J Med 2001;344(19):1434–41.

32. Miller P, Hattersley G, Riis B, et al. Effect of abaloparatide vs placebo on new vertebral fractures in postmenopausal women with osteoporosis: a randomized clinical trial. JAMA 2016;316(7):722–33.

33. Cosman F, Crittenden DB, Adachi JD, et al. Romosozumab treatment in postmenopausal women with osteoporosis. N Engl J Med 2016;375(16):1532–43.

34. Saag KG, Petersen J, Brandi ML, et al. Romosozumab or alendronate for fracture prevention in women with osteoporosis. N Engl J Med 2017;377(15):1417–27.

35. McClung MR, Grauer A, Boonen S, et al. Romosozumab in postmenopausal women with low bone mineral density. N Engl J Med 2014;370(5):412–20.

36. Cummings SR, McCulloch C. Explanations for the difference in rates of cardiovascular events in a trial of alendronate and romosozumab. Osteoporos Int 2020;31(6):1019–21.

37. Kendler DL, Marin F, Zerbini CAF, et al. Effects of teriparatide and risedronate on new fractures in post-menopausal women with severe osteoporosis (VERO): a multicentre, double-blind, double-dummy, randomised controlled trial. Lancet 2018;391(10117):230–40.

38. Vilaca T, Schini M, Harnan S, et al. The risk of hip and non-vertebral fractures in type 1 and type 2 diabetes: a systematic review and meta-analysis update. Bone 2020;137:115457.

39. Khan KS, Andersen H. The impact of diabetic neuropathy on activities of daily living, postural balance and risk of falls - a systematic review. J Diabetes Sci Technol 2021;16(2):289–94.

40. Hidayat K, Fang QL, Shi BM, et al. Influence of glycemic control and hypoglycemia on the risk of fracture in patients with diabetes mellitus: a systematic review and meta-analysis of observational studies. Osteoporos Int 2021;32(9):1693–704.

41. Díez-Pérez A, Marin F, Eriksen EF, et al. Effects of teriparatide on hip and upper limb fractures in patients with osteoporosis: a systematic review and meta-analysis. Bone 2019;120:1–8.

42. Eriksen EF, Keaveny TM, Gallagher ER, et al. Literature review: the effects of teriparatide therapy at the hip in patients with osteoporosis. Bone 2014;67:246–56.

43. Johansson H, Siggeirsdóttir K, Harvey NC, et al. Imminent risk of fracture after fracture. Osteoporos Int 2017;28(3):775–80.

44. Unson CG, Siccion E, Gaztambide J, et al. Nonadherence and osteoporosis treatment preferences of older women: a qualitative study. J Women's Health (2002) 2003;12(10):1037–45.

45. Reid IR, Horne AM, Mihov B, et al. Fracture prevention with zoledronate in older women with osteopenia. N Engl J Med 2018;379(25):2407–16.

46. Grey A, Bolland MJ, Horne A, et al. Five years of anti-resorptive activity after a single dose of zoledronate — results from a randomized double-blind placebo-controlled trial. Bone 2012;50(6):1389–93.

47. Grey A, Horne A, Gamble G, et al. Ten years of very infrequent zoledronate therapy in older women: an open-label extension of a randomized trial. J Clin Endocrinol Metab 2020;105(4):dgaa062.

Polypharmacy in the Emergency Department

Khai H. Nguyen, MD, MHS[a],*, Vaishal Tolia, MD, MPH[b], Laura A. Hart, PharmD, MS[c]

KEYWORDS

- Polypharmacy • Adverse drug events • Potentially inappropriate medications
- Medication reconciliation

KEY POINTS

- Adults aged 75 years and older use the emergency department (ED) at higher rates than other segments of the adult population.
- Adverse drug events (ADEs) are a consequence of polypharmacy, and the use of potentially inappropriate medications (PIMs) contributes to an increased risk of ADEs.
- Accurate medication list through medication reconciliation allows for conducting an effective medication review, which can identify various medication-related problems and help to optimize medication prescribing.
- Implicit and explicit tools help to optimize prescribing as well as reducing older adults' exposure to PIMs and adverse medication-related outcomes.
- Deprescribing in the ED can be challenging because it requires medication adjustments, as well as ongoing support and follow-up. However, if a medication is actively causing harm or presenting a safety concern, discontinuation, dose adjustment, or a temporary hold may be necessary.

INTRODUCTION

Every care setting is influenced by the demographic shift of the aging population. The emergency department (ED) is no exception, with adults aged 75 years and older using the ED at higher rates than other segments of the adult population. Moreover, the ED is the frontline for all aging-related ailments and a cauldron for brewing risk factors and sentinel events to boil over culminating in morbidity and mortality. Older adults presenting to the ED often have multiple complex medical and social conditions and take numerous medications. The sheer number of older adults flowing through

[a] Department of Medicine, University of California, 8899 University Center Lane, Suite 400, MC 0877, San Diego, CA 92122, USA; [b] Department of Emergency Medicine, University of California, San Diego, 200 West Arbor Drive, MC 8676, San Diego, CA 92103, USA; [c] Skaggs School of Pharmacy and Pharmaceutical Sciences, University of California, San Diego, 9500 Gilman Drive, MC 0657, La Jolla, CA 92093, USA
* Corresponding author.
E-mail address: khn059@health.ucsd.edu
Twitter: @laura_a_hart (L.A.H.)

Clin Geriatr Med 38 (2022) 727–732
https://doi.org/10.1016/j.cger.2022.05.012
0749-0690/22/© 2022 Elsevier Inc. All rights reserved.

EDs worldwide commands attention toward medications alongside the myriad of other challenges posed in this most acute of care settings.

Emergent medical conditions often threaten an older person's usual state of health in such a way that interrupts their homeostasis and renders them vulnerable to the very medications they often rely on to maintain their well-being. With an older person's health spiraling into a maelstrom of morbid uncertainty, the concern for polypharmacy rises to the top because this issue can contribute to adverse drug events (ADEs), drug interactions, and the introduction of potentially inappropriate medications (PIMs), particularly in the acute care setting of the ED.

The American College of Emergency Physicians (ACEP) instituted an accreditation process to recognize the various levels of geriatric emergency departments (GEDs) and recognized the use of workflows and protocols to identify, screen, and engage a cadre of emergency practitioners to address polypharmacy at time when older patients are most susceptible to adverse outcomes.[1] Further, ACEP, alongside the American Geriatrics Society, Emergency Nurses Association, and the Society for Academic Emergency Medicine, developed GED guidelines.[2] GEDs serve as an aspirational solution to address the challenges that afflict older adults and health systems. With education, training, protocols, and emphasis on the team-based approach to the comprehensive care of older adults in the ED, this model exemplifies a specific pathway to evaluate and manage geriatric syndromes both for early identification and prevention, as well as at extreme decompensation. Among these geriatric syndromes is polypharmacy. Although not all EDs are accredited as GEDs, the workflows and protocols in place within GEDs can serve as important guidance for EDs in the care of older adults.

Arrival to an ED can often be for serious and life-threatening conditions involving pain, trauma, infections, bleeding, dyspnea among an array of acute presentations that can be further complicated by hemodynamic instability, cardiovascular compromise, dehydration, acute kidney and/or hepatic injury, and central nervous system malfunction. Polypharmacy undoubtedly compounds these factors and can detrimentally affect the older individual's health outcome depending on the mix of medications, potential interactions, and ADEs. This challenge in ED care also presents an opportunity to reconcile medications, screen for potential interactions, avoid the pitfalls of inappropriate medication use, and even deprescribe drugs when indicated. The care setting that is the ED and the dire situation that is a medical emergency is a critical juncture for these life-saving interventions to occur or the alternative, allowing the complications to manifest in such a way that fosters further morbidity and mortality.

DISCUSSION
Adverse Drug Events and Potentially Inappropriate Medications

ADEs, which refer to injuries resulting from medication use, are an important consequence of polypharmacy.[3] The prevalence of ED visits for ADEs in the United States is estimated to be 4 per 1000.[4] Among older adults, anticoagulants, antidiabetic medications, and opioids are involved in more than half of ED visits attributable to ADEs.[4] Further, the use of PIMs contributes to an increased risk of ADEs.[5] PIMs are medications where the risk of harm outweighs potential benefits, notably in older adults (**Table 1**).[6] Various tools exist to identify PIMS, as discussed in the subsection "Tools to Optimize Prescribing" below.

MEDICATION RECONCILIATION AND REVIEW

Medication reconciliation refers to the process of creating an accurate list of all medications a patient is taking at home and updating the medical record accordingly.[7] In

Table 1
Examples of PIMs and potential risks

Medication Class	Potential Risks
NSAIDs	Gastrointestinal bleeding, kidney damage, increased blood pressure
Anticholinergics	Confusion, sedation, blurred vision, constipation
Benzodiazepines and z-drugs	Delirium, falls
Long-acting sulfonylureas	Hypoglycemia

Abbreviation: NSAIDs, nonsteroidal anti-inflammatory drugs.

addition to prescription medications, medication reconciliation should include over-the-counter medications and supplements. Another important, but sometimes overlooked, piece of medication reconciliation is documenting a patient's allergies. Performing effective medication reconciliation is imperative for ensuring appropriate medication use, preventing medication errors, and decreasing the risk of ADEs through transitions of care.

Medication reconciliation in the ED may be conducted by nurses, physicians, or pharmacy staff. In recent years, many studies have evaluated pharmacy-led medication reconciliation efforts in the ED setting and have found that medication reconciliation conducted by pharmacists or pharmacy technicians leads to a greater reduction in medication discrepancies as compared with medication reconciliation conducted by other health-care professionals.[8] Not all EDs have dedicated pharmacy staff or enough resources to screen all older adults presenting to the ED.

Medication reconciliation in the ED has implications in the context of (1) evaluating and initiating medications in the ED, (2) discharging a patient home from the ED with new prescription medications, and (3) admitting a patient to the hospital from the ED. Collecting an accurate medication history through medication reconciliation is a crucial step to shed light on drug-related impact on a patient's presenting chief complaint. For example, if an older adult presents to the ED with altered mental status, identifying potential medication-related causes is imperative. In addition, collecting updated allergy information as part of medication reconciliation is critical in avoiding an allergic reaction to medications administered in the ED or prescribed on discharge from the ED. Further, collecting an accurate medication list can help to avoid a potential drug–drug interaction for medications administered in the ED or prescribed on discharge from the ED. Further, conducting effective medication reconciliation in the ED can help to avoid medication-related problems on admission to the hospital from the ED, for example, by ensuring medications for chronic conditions are documented and ordered as appropriate in the acute inpatient setting. Further, inappropriate prescribing that occurs resulting from improper medication reconciliation has the potential to be carried over through transitions of care and subsequently have ongoing implications for patient safety.

Examples of potential situations that can result from incomplete or ineffective medication reconciliation in the ED are provided below:

Patient has allergy to morphine with anaphylactic reaction that is not documented during medication reconciliation → Patient administered morphine in the ED and experiences anaphylaxis.

Regular use of over-the-counter ibuprofen is not documented during medication reconciliation → Patient prescribed indomethacin on ED discharge without counseling to hold ibuprofen and subsequently experiences gastrointestinal bleeding from using 2 nonsteroidal anti-inflammatory drugs concurrently.

Use of the antiseizure medication levetiracetam is not documented during medication reconciliation → Patient is not ordered levetiracetam on hospital admission and experiences a seizure.

Ultimately, collecting an accurate medication list through medication reconciliation allows for conducting an effective medication review. A medication review can identify various medication-related problems and help to optimize medication prescribing. Medication-related problems can be classified into the broad categories of untreated condition, medication without indication, improper medication selection (eg, PIMs), subtherapeutic dosage, supratherapeutic dosage, therapeutic duplication, adverse drug reactions, and drug interactions.

TOOLS TO ADDRESS POLYPHARMACY AND OPTIMIZE PRESCRIBING

Various tools exist for ED clinicians to use when addressing polypharmacy and ensuring appropriate prescribing in older adults. These tools can be classified as explicit or implicit. Explicit tools are criterion-based, whereas implicit tools are judgment-based.

Explicit Tools

Examples of explicit tools to optimize prescribing are Beers Criteria[6] and STOPP/START (Screening Tool of Older People's Prescriptions [STOPP] and Screening Tool to Alert to Right Treatment [START]) criteria.[9] The Beers Criteria were originally developed in 1991 by physician Mark Beers, MD, and have subsequently been updated with the most recent update in 2019 by the American Geriatrics Society. With an overarching goal of reducing older adults' exposure to PIMs, aims of the Beers Criteria include improving medication selection in older adults, educating clinicians and patients, and reducing adverse medication-related outcomes in older adults. The criteria are intended for use in older adults across care settings, with the important exceptions of hospice care and palliative care. The most recent revision of the Beers Criteria outlines medications that should be:

Avoided in most older adults.

Avoided in older adults with specific health conditions.

Avoided in combination with other medications because of the risk of harmful drug–drug interactions.

Used with caution because of the potential for harmful side effects.

Dosed differently or avoided in older adults who have reduced kidney function.

STOPP/START criteria were originally developed in Europe in 2008 and most recently updated in 2015. Similar to the Beers Criteria, the STOPP criteria address PIMs, whereas the START criteria address potential prescribing omissions. The STOPP/START tool consists of 80 criteria within STOPP and 34 criteria within START.

Implicit Tools

A prominent example of an implicit tool to optimize prescribing is the Medication Appropriateness Index (MAI).[10,11] The MAI consists of 10 questions to ask when evaluating the appropriateness of a particular medication in a given patient. Although this tool may be cumbersome to use, it can provide an important framework to use during the medication review process. It can be especially helpful for targeting unnecessary medication use, thereby addressing the issue of polypharmacy. It can also help to optimize medication use in various other ways, which are outlined in the questions included in the MAI shown below:

Is there an indication for the drug?

Is the medication effective for the condition?
Is the dosage correct?
Are the directions correct?
Are the directions practical?
Are there clinically significant drug–drug interactions?
Are there clinically significant drug–disease/condition interactions?
Is there unnecessary duplication with other drug(s)?
Is the duration of therapy acceptable?
Is this drug the least expensive alternative compared with others of equal utility?

ELECTRONIC MEDICAL RECORDS

Electronic medical records (EMRs) are now widely used by health systems. EMRs can help to optimize medication prescribing in the ED through embedded clinical decision support tools. These tools can provide real-time alert to the prescriber of the presence of PIMs, as well as alternative medications that would be both safe and effective. These tools can also alert clinicians to the appropriate dose of a medication in certain settings, such as kidney impairment. Further, reports can be generated for individual prescribers to show medication prescribing patterns over time and allow for further pertinent education to be provided to optimize prescribing.

DEPRESCRIBING AND DE-ESCALATING MEDICATION THERAPY

Deprescribing refers to the systematic process of medication withdrawal, through either discontinuing medications or reducing medication doses, under the guidance and supervision of a health-care professional.[12] Goals of deprescribing include reducing medication burden, decreasing fall risk, improving cognition, and reducing risk of hospitalization and death. Deprescribing is an important way to reduce polypharmacy and improve health outcomes in older adults.[13]

Deprescribing in the ED presents inherent challenges given the short-term nature of contact between the patient and clinicians in this setting. Deprescribing often requires medication tapering, as well as clinician support and follow-up. Further, patients often receive outpatient prescriptions from health systems that are disparate in their records and do not participate in health information exchange. This makes deprescribing (either dose adjustment or discontinuation) a greater challenge. Not knowing the history behind a long-term medication also gives pause to the ED team in making drastic changes to the medication list during the ED encounter. However, if a medication is actively causing harm or presenting a safety concern, discontinuation, dose adjustment, or a temporary hold may be necessary.

CLINICS CARE POINTS

- Performing effective medication reconciliation in the emergency department (ED) is imperative for ensuring appropriate medication use, preventing medication errors, and decreasing the risk of adverse drug events through transitions of care.

- Several tools exist for ED clinicians to use when addressing polypharmacy and ensuring appropriate prescribing in older adults, including Beers Criteria, STOPP/START (Screening Tool of Older People's Prescriptions [STOPP] and Screening Tool to Alert to Right Treatment [START]) criteria, and the Medication Appropriateness Index.

- Deprescribing or de-escalating medications in the ED setting presents challenges given the short-term nature of contact between the patient and ED clinicians. Consideration of such processes should generally be undertaken in the outpatient continuity of care. However, discontinuing a medication in the ED may be warranted in specific cases.

DISCLOSURE

The authors have nothing to disclose.

REFERENCES

1. Huff C. ACEP accrediting geriatric emergency departments: Move to Standardize special Needs elder care. Ann Emerg Med 2018;71(5):A21–4.
2. Carpenter CR, Bromley M, Caterino JM, et al, ACEP Geriatric Emergency Medicine Section, American Geriatrics Society, Emergency Nurses Association, and Society for Academic Emergency Medicine Academy of Geriatric Emergency Medicine. Optimal older adult emergency care: introducing multidisciplinary geriatric emergency department guidelines from the American College of emergency physicians, American geriatrics Society, emergency nurses association, and Society for Academic emergency medicine. J Am Geriatr Soc 2014;62(7):1360–3.
3. Institute of Medicine. Preventing medication errors. Washington, DC: National Academies Press; 2006.
4. Shehab N, Lovegrove MC, Geller AI, et al. US emergency department visits for outpatient Adverse drug events, 2013-2014. JAMA 2016;316(20):2115–25.
5. Xing XX, Zhu C, Liang HY, et al. Associations between potentially inappropriate medications and adverse health outcomes in the elderly: a systematic review and meta-analysis. Ann Pharmacother 2019;53(10):1005–19.
6. 2019 American geriatrics Society Beers Criteria® update expert Panel. American geriatrics Society 2019 updated AGS Beers Criteria® for potentially inappropriate medication Use in older adults. J Am Geriatr Soc 2019;67(4):674–94.
7. Medication reconciliation to prevent adverse drug events. Institute for Healthcare Improvement website. Available at: http://www.ihi.org/Topics/ADEsMedication Reconciliation/Pages/default.aspx. Accessed February 20, 2022.
8. Choi YJ, Kim H. Effect of pharmacy-led medication reconciliation in emergency departments: a systematic review and meta-analysis. J Clin Pharm Ther 2019; 44(6):932–45.
9. O'Mahony D, O'Sullivan D, Byrne S, et al. STOPP/START criteria for potentially inappropriate prescribing in older people: version 2. Age Ageing 2015;44(2): 213–8 [published correction appears in Age Ageing. 2018 May 1;47(3):489].
10. Hanlon JT, Schmader KE, Samsa GP, et al. A method for assessing drug therapy appropriateness. J Clin Epidemiol 1992;45(10):1045–51.
11. Samsa GP, Hanlon JT, Schmader KE, et al. A summated score for the medication appropriateness index: development and assessment of clinimetric properties including content validity. J Clin Epidemiol 1994;47(8):891–6.
12. Reeve E, Shakib S, Hendrix I, et al. Review of deprescribing processes and development of an evidence-based, patient-centered deprescribing process. Br J Clin Pharmacol 2014;78:738–47.
13. Scott IA, Hilmer SN, Reeve E, et al. Reducing inappropriate polypharmacy: the process of deprescribing. JAMA Intern Med 2015;175(5):827–34.

UNITED STATES POSTAL SERVICE ®
Statement of Ownership, Management, and Circulation
(All Periodicals Publications Except Requester Publications)

1. Publication Title	2. Publication Number	3. Filing Date
CLINICS IN GERIATRIC MEDICINE	000 – 704	9/18/2022

4. Issue Frequency	5. Number of Issues Published Annually	6. Annual Subscription Price
FEB, MAY, AUG, NOV	4	$303.00

7. Complete Mailing Address of Known Office of Publication (Not printer) (Street, city, county, state, and ZIP+4®)

ELSEVIER INC.
230 Park Avenue, Suite 800
New York, NY 10169

Contact Person
Malathi Samayan

Telephone (Include area code)
91-44-4299-4507

8. Complete Mailing Address of Headquarters or General Business Office of Publisher (Not printer)

ELSEVIER INC.
230 Park Avenue, Suite 800
New York, NY 10169

9. Full Names and Complete Mailing Addresses of Publisher, Editor, and Managing Editor (Do not leave blank)

Publisher (Name and complete mailing address)

DOLORES MELONI, ELSEVIER INC.
1600 JOHN F KENNEDY BLVD. SUITE 1800
PHILADELPHIA, PA 19103-2899

Editor (Name and complete mailing address)

TAYLOR HAYES, ELSEVIER INC.
1600 JOHN F KENNEDY BLVD. SUITE 1800
PHILADELPHIA, PA 19103-2899

Managing Editor (Name and complete mailing address)

PATRICK MANLEY, ELSEVIER INC.
1600 JOHN F KENNEDY BLVD. SUITE 1800
PHILADELPHIA, PA 19103-2899

10. Owner (Do not leave blank. If the publication is owned by a corporation, give the name and address of the corporation immediately followed by the names and addresses of all stockholders owning or holding 1 percent or more of the total amount of stock. If not owned by a corporation, give the names and addresses of the individual owners. If owned by a partnership or other unincorporated firm, give its name and address as well as those of each individual owner. If the publication is published by a nonprofit organization, give its name and address.)

Full Name	Complete Mailing Address
WHOLLY OWNED SUBSIDIARY OF REED/ELSEVIER, US HOLDINGS	1600 JOHN F KENNEDY BLVD. SUITE 1800 PHILADELPHIA, PA 19103-2899

11. Known Bondholders, Mortgagees, and Other Security Holders Owning or Holding 1 Percent or More of Total Amount of Bonds, Mortgages, or Other Securities. If none, check box ► ☑ None

Full Name	Complete Mailing Address
N/A	

12. Tax Status (For completion by nonprofit organizations authorized to mail at nonprofit rates) (Check one)
The purpose, function, and nonprofit status of this organization and the exempt status for federal income tax purposes:
☒ Has Not Changed During Preceding 12 Months
☐ Has Changed During Preceding 12 Months (Publisher must submit explanation of change with this statement)

PS Form **3526**, July 2014 [Page 1 of 4 (see instructions page 4)] PSN: 7530-01-000-9931 PRIVACY NOTICE: See our privacy policy on www.usps.com.

13. Publication Title	14. Issue Date for Circulation Data Below
CLINICS IN GERIATRIC MEDICINE	MAY 2022

15. Extent and Nature of Circulation			Average No. Copies Each Issue During Preceding 12 Months	No. Copies of Single Issue Published Nearest to Filing Date
a. Total Number of Copies (Net press run)			143	122
b. Paid Circulation (By Mail and Outside the Mail)	(1)	Mailed Outside-County Paid Subscriptions Stated on PS Form 3541 (Include paid distribution above nominal rate, advertiser's proof copies, and exchange copies)	69	65
	(2)	Mailed In-County Paid Subscriptions Stated on PS Form 3541 (Include paid distribution above nominal rate, advertiser's proof copies, and exchange copies)	0	0
	(3)	Paid Distribution Outside the Mails Including Sales Through Dealers and Carriers, Street Vendors, Counter Sales, and Other Paid Distribution Outside USPS®	31	29
	(4)	Paid Distribution by Other Classes of Mail Through the USPS (e.g. First-Class Mail®)	0	0
c. Total Paid Distribution (Sum of 15b (1), (2), (3), and (4)) ►			100	94
d. Free or Nominal Rate Distribution (By Mail and Outside the Mail)	(1)	Free or Nominal Rate Outside-County Copies included on PS Form 3541	29	11
	(2)	Free or Nominal Rate In-County Copies Included on PS Form 3541	0	0
	(3)	Free or Nominal Rate Copies Mailed at Other Classes Through the USPS (e.g. First-Class Mail)	0	0
	(4)	Free or Nominal Rate Distribution Outside the Mail (Carriers or other means)	0	0
e. Total Free or Nominal Rate Distribution (Sum of 15d (1), (2), (3) and (4)) ►			29	11
f. Total Distribution (Sum of 15c and 15e) ►			129	105
g. Copies not Distributed (See Instructions to Publishers #4 (page 43)) ►			14	17
h. Total (Sum of 15f and g) ►			143	122
i. Percent Paid (15c divided by 15f times 100) ►			77.51%	89.52%

* If you are claiming electronic copies, go to line 16 on page 3. If you are not claiming electronic copies, skip to line 17 on page 3.

PS Form **3526**, July 2014 (Page 2 of 4)

16. Electronic Copy Circulation	Average No. Copies Each Issue During Preceding 12 Months	No. Copies of Single Issue Published Nearest to Filing Date
a. Paid Electronic Copies ►		
b. Total Paid Print Copies (Line 15c) + Paid Electronic Copies (Line 16a) ►		
c. Total Print Distribution (Line 15f) + Paid Electronic Copies (Line 16a) ►		
d. Percent Paid (Both Print & Electronic Copies) (16b divided by 16c × 100) ►		

☒ I certify that 50% of all my distributed copies (electronic and print) are paid above a nominal price.

17. Publication of Statement of Ownership

☒ If the publication is a general publication, publication of this statement is required. Will be printed
in the NOVEMBER 2022 issue of this publication.

☐ Publication not required.

18. Signature and Title of Editor, Publisher, Business Manager or Owner

Malathi Samayan — Malathi Samayan - Distribution Controller

Date: 9/18/2022

I certify that all information furnished on this form is true and complete. I understand that anyone who furnishes false or misleading information on this form or who omits material or information requested on the form may be subject to criminal sanctions (including fines and imprisonment) and/or civil sanctions (including civil penalties).

PS Form **3526**, July 2014 (Page 3 of 4) PRIVACY NOTICE: See our privacy policy on www.usps.com

Printed and bound by CPI Group (UK) Ltd, Croydon, CR0 4YY

03/10/2024

01040470-0011